Provider-Based Entities:
A Guide to Regulatory and Billing Compliance

Gina M. Reese, Esq., RN

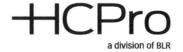

Provider-Based Entities: A Guide to Regulatory and Billing Compliance is published by HCPro, a division of BLR.

Copyright © 2015 HCPro, a division of BLR

All rights reserved. Printed in the United States of America.   5   4   3   2   1

Download the additional materials of this book at *www.hcpro.com/downloads/12439*

ISBN: 978-1-55645-715-9

No part of this publication may be reproduced, in any form or by any means, without prior written consent of HCPro or the Copyright Clearance Center (978-750-8400). Please notify us immediately if you have received an unauthorized copy.

HCPro provides information resources for the healthcare industry.

HCPro is not affiliated in any way with The Joint Commission, which owns the JCAHO and Joint Commission trademarks.

Gina M. Reese, Esq., RN, Author
Jaclyn Fitzgerald, Editor
Melissa Osborn, Product Director
Erin Callahan, Vice President, Product Development & Content Strategy
Elizabeth Petersen, Executive Vice President, Healthcare
Matt Sharpe, Production Supervisor
Vincent Skyers, Design Manager
Vicki McMahan, Sr. Graphic Designer/Layout
Jason Gregory, Cover Designer

Advice given is general. Readers should consult professional counsel for specific legal, ethical, or clinical questions.

Arrangements can be made for quantity discounts. For more information, contact:

HCPro
100 Winners Circle, Suite 300
Brentwood, TN 37027
Telephone: 800-650-6787 or 781-639-1872
Fax: 800-785-9212
Email: *customerservice@hcpro.com*

Visit HCPro online at:
www.hcpro.com and *www.hcmarketplace.com*

Table of Contents

About the Author

Gina M. Reese, Esq., RN, is an expert in Medicare rules and regulations and is an instructor for HCPro's Medicare Boot Camp—Hospital Version® and Medicare Boot Camp—Utilization Review Version®. As a registered nurse and attorney, Reese has specialized for nearly 30 years in assisting healthcare providers in survey preparation, compliance with Medicare certification and Joint Commission accreditation requirements, responses to adverse certification/accreditation findings, appeals of reimbursement disputes, and representation in fraud/abuse investigations and disclosures.

Reese graduated *magna cum laude* from Whittier College School of Law in Los Angeles after receiving a bachelor's degree in business administration with an emphasis in accounting, *magna cum laude* from California State University at Los Angeles, and with a nursing degree from Samuel Merritt Hospital School of Nursing in Oakland, California. After earning her nursing degree, Reese chose to specialize in pediatric intensive care and special procedure unit services in chemotherapy and diabetic care/education at University Hospital in San Diego and Children's Hospital at Los Angeles (CHLA). She then moved into a position as supervisor in utilization management and quality review at CHLA, overseeing a cadre of nurses performing these tasks, staffing peer review and quality committees at the hospital, and drafting and managing policies and procedures for these activities. While attending law school, Reese accepted a senior level position at Shriners Hospital for Crippled Children, Los Angeles, as the director of risk management, quality assurance, and utilization management.

After completing law school, Reese worked for 10 years as an associate attorney and later a partner at Hooper, Lundy, and Bookman, a boutique health law firm in Century City, California, representing healthcare providers across the country. For the subsequent 10 years, Reese worked as senior counsel at Kaiser Foundation Health Plan/Hospitals, further broadening her knowledge of healthcare law to include managed healthcare, provider contracting, Medicare Advantage (including risk adjustment), revenue cycle, coding, privacy, electronic health records, and many other areas. Reese is now the risk manager at Methodist Hospital of Southern California, responding to patient grievances and adverse events, and leading the hospital's enterprise risk management program.

Reese's extensive experience in the health law field allows her to furnish consulting advice that prospectively takes into account the full breadth of the clinical, regulatory, fraud and abuse, coding, and reimbursement needs of clients. This includes development and maintenance of educational materials and presentations, risk management, compliance programs and tools, policies and procedures, auditing processes, documentation review, and coordination with coding, claim submission, revenue cycle, and reimbursement.

Billing for Provider-Based Entities: The Big Picture

1

Introduction

You have just taken a job as the hospital's new revenue cycle leader after years of toiling away as a billing coordinator. One of your employees comes to you and states that she wonders whether the hospital is in compliance with the Medicare provider-based billing rules. Puzzled, you ask her where she heard this term. She states that her friends who work at a nearby hospital told her that the Medicare Administrative Contractor (MAC) is auditing that hospital for compliance with these rules in their infusion clinic.

You begin to panic. Do you or your coworkers know whether your hospital is in compliance? How do you go about auditing for compliance? Who is responsible—is it you? Why would this apply to an infusion clinic? What else do you not know?

Relax—billing for provider-based entities is not rocket science! Chances are you already know more than you think you do. Most provider-based billing concepts are commonsensical and based on big-picture concepts that you already know. However, you should pay attention to the details covered in the remaining chapters of this book and ensure compliance with them. There is a lot of evidence that the Centers for Medicare and Medicaid Services (CMS) and the Department of Health and Human Services (HHS) Office of Inspector General (OIG) are increasing their scrutiny of compliance with these requirements. In addition, failure to be in compliance could be very costly and more time-consuming in the long run than auditing the hospital's state of compliance now. For example, in the six months from October 2014 to April 2015 alone, two hospitals—W.A. Foote Memorial Hospital in Michigan and Our Lady of Lourdes Memorial Hospital in New York—have self-disclosed and settled cases with the federal government for overpayments related to provider-based billing of $3.3 million and $2.6 million, respectively (Settlement

Agreement between United States of America and Our Lady of Lourdes Memorial Hospital, 2014; Provider-Based Rules Trigger, 2015).

More investigations and repayments are likely to follow in the coming months and years, given the new tools being implemented in 2015 and 2016 to more readily identify provider-based clinics.

We will go into great detail about all of the requirements in the following chapters, but it is helpful to first see the forest through the trees. The following is a summary of the big picture regarding billing for provider-based entities.

What Is a Provider-Based Department?

Provider-based billing is conducted by "main providers." For Medicare purposes, a main provider is defined as any provider that either creates or acquires ownership of another entity to deliver additional healthcare services under the name, ownership, and financial and administrative control of the hospital (42 *CFR* §413.65[a][2]). While main providers include more than hospitals, the vast majority of provider-based entities are owned and operated by acute care hospitals and critical access hospitals (CAH). Therefore, we will primarily refer to hospitals as the main providers when we are discussing these requirements in this book.

Most simply put, provider-based departments are the locations where main providers furnish services to their own outpatients, as well as some remote locations and satellite facilities where hospitals furnish inpatient services. These locations are subservient and responsible to the hospital for all purposes, including oversight, control, clinical care, licensing, accreditation, and Medicare certification. Just like the main hospital, they must meet specific CMS requirements; these requirements are more onerous for provider-based departments located more than 250 yards off of the hospital campus (off-campus departments). We will interchangeably refer to "provider-based" and "hospital-based" when referring to the entities operated by main providers, since most provider-based entities are operated by hospitals. We may also interchangeably refer to provider-based "departments" in the upcoming chapters as "clinics," "entities," "settings," and "locations." Provider-based departments are not the same as freestanding physician offices or other entities that are separately licensed, accredited, or certified, even if those entities are located close to the hospital, furnish outpatient services to the same population of patients, and/or are owned by the hospital. The difference is that freestanding entities are considered to furnish their clinical services independent of the hospital and are responsible for independently meeting their own licensing and regulatory requirements.

Billing and Reimbursement for Provider-Based Departments

As part of the hospital, services furnished in provider-based departments must be billed to Medicare and other government payers as services of the main provider. Billing for provider-based departments is generally accomplished through submission of two claim forms: one for the facility component and one for the professional component of the services.

The main provider (e.g., hospital) bills for the facility component of the services furnished in these provider-based departments on the (ASC) X12N 837I (Institutional) Version 5010A2 electronic claim form (837I) or UB-04 Uniform Bill paper claim under its own name and provider number, and it claims the costs for these locations on its own Medicare and Medicaid cost report. The coding for these services is no different than other hospital outpatient services, except for the newest requirement that the hospital must use the modifier "-PO" on each line item for services furnished in off-campus provider-based departments.

The professional component of the services furnished in these locations is billed on a separate (ASC) X12N 837P (Professional) Version 5010A1 electronic billing form (837P) or CMS-1500 paper claim form (CMS-1500), using the standard Current Procedural Terminology (CPT®) codes for professional services. These services are billed by the physician or nonphysician practitioner (NPP) under the name and national payment identifier of the professional (or medical group) with the appropriate place of service (POS) code to show CMS that the services were furnished in a hospital outpatient department. Historically, professional services furnished to hospital outpatients in all provider-based departments would be billed using a POS of "22." However, CMS redefined POS 22 in *Transmittal 3315*, dated August 6, 2015. Effective January 1, 2016, POS 22 is to be used for professional services furnished to hospital outpatients only when the services are furnished on the main hospital campus (within 250 yards of the main hospital buildings). In the same transmittal, CMS introduced POS "19," which is to be used to bill professional services furnished to hospital outpatients in off-campus provider-based departments, effective January 1, 2016.

In contrast, billing for services furnished in freestanding physician offices is performed strictly using one CMS-1500 claim form for the global service under the name and identifiers of the professional or medical group operating the clinic. These claims are submitted with the POS code that identifies these services as being provided in the freestanding physician office (POS "11"). Separately certified entities and facilities (e.g., home health agencies [HHA], skilled nursing facilities [SNF]) are billed separately from the hospital claim form on the billing form appropriate for that type of facility and under that entity's provider/supplier number and name.

Reimbursement for Services at Provider-Based Entities

Services furnished by physicians and NPPs in freestanding physician offices and billed on the CMS-1500 form are paid to the professionals based on the Medicare physician fee schedule (MPFS). Because the physician is in effect billing globally for the entire service (both the facility and professional component of the service), he or she receives the entire fee schedule amount for the service.

In contrast, services furnished in provider-based departments are reimbursed separately to the professional and the main provider. The main provider (e.g., hospital) is paid only for the facility component of the services, which is billed on the UB-04 claim form. The facility component is intended to reimburse the hospital for the services of the hospital staff, supplies, and overhead necessary to operate the clinic and furnish the services.

The hands-on professional services of physicians and NPPs furnished to the patients in provider-based departments (billed on the CMS-1500 form) are still paid separately to the physicians/ NPPs based on the MPFS. However, the physicians are paid a reduced portion of the MPFS amount to account for the fact that the services were furnished in the hospital outpatient department, rather than in the physician's office setting.

If you add up the facility payment made to the hospital and the professional fee paid to the physician, the total payment made by Medicare for services furnished in provider-based departments (the facility plus the professional components) has historically been higher in provider-based departments as compared to the payment made for the same service furnished in a freestanding facility. This increased overall payment is attributable to a higher payment to the hospital (the physician's payment is actually reduced under this system) and is designed to compensate the hospital for the higher overhead costs required to operate as the main provider, which is subject to more regulations than the freestanding physician clinic locations.

This increased reimbursement for services furnished in provider-based departments may be changing under the increased packaging concepts required under the hospital outpatient prospective payment system (OPPS), which mandates a single packaged reimbursement for clinic and emergency room visits and all related ancillary services. However, this likely comes too late to halt the increased scrutiny CMS has planned for provider-based departments, especially for off-campus departments, due to the historical criticism of this reimbursement by the Medicare Payment Advisory Committee (MedPac), the OIG, and the public, as discussed later.

Patient Cost-Sharing and Deductibles in Provider-Based Departments

Medicare beneficiaries are charged a monthly premium for Part B services in addition to a small annual deductible. This deductible does not vary based on whether the beneficiary seeks services in a freestanding physician office or in a provider-based department.

Medicare beneficiaries are also liable for a coinsurance or copayment equal to approximately 20% of the Medicare allowable amount for each covered Part B service, with some exceptions. Beneficiaries who receive medical services at freestanding physician offices generally only incur liability for one copayment for the visit. This cost-sharing is based on the Medicare-allowed amount paid to the physician for these services.

In contrast, patients who seek the exact same services in a provider-based department receive bills for two copayments: one from the physician for the professional component of the services and the other from the hospital for the facility component of the services. The total amount paid by Medicare to the physician and the hospital for these services is generally higher in a provider-based department than the total amount that would have been paid for these services in the freestanding physician office. Therefore, the beneficiary's liability for these services is also generally higher than the cost-sharing they would have been subjected to for these services at a freestanding physician office. On top of that, this increase is more obvious to the beneficiaries because they receive two separate bills from the hospital and the physician.

Why the Government Is Concerned About Provider-Based Billing

Hospitals originated primarily to furnish inpatient services, since there were few outpatient services available other than minor treatments, dressings, and medications, and these services were primarily furnished in community physician offices and in the home. However, as technology has advanced, more complex outpatient medical services have become available, and these services have increasingly been provided in hospital outpatient departments.

The use of hospital-based clinics has rapidly increased in the past several years, as hospitals and physicians have recognized the advantages of vertically integrating their services. MedPac analyzes Medicare spending for various types of services, as well as beneficiary access to services, in its annual review of each of the updated Medicare payment policy regulations. In its 2015 Report to Congress, MedPac examined the increasing shift of Medicare spending from freestanding physician offices to hospital outpatient departments:

"From 2012 to 2013, the use of outpatient services increased by 3.8 percent per Medicare FFS Part B beneficiary; over the past seven years, the cumulative increase was 33 percent. Roughly one-third of the growth in outpatient volume in 2013 was due to a 10 percent increase in the number of evaluation and management (E/M) visits billed as [hospital] outpatient services. This growth in part reflects hospitals purchasing freestanding physician practices and converting them into hospital outpatient departments (HOPDs). As hospitals do so, market share shifts from freestanding physician offices to HOPDs ... From 2012 to 2013, hospital-based E/M visits per beneficiary grew by 9.4 percent compared with 1.1 percent growth in physician-office-based visits.

Other categories of services are also shifting to the higher cost site of care, such as echocardiograms and nuclear cardiology. Hospital-based echocardiograms per capita grew by 7.4 percent compared with an 8.0 percent decline in physician-office echocardiograms. Nuclear cardiology grew by 0.4 percent in HOPDs compared with a 12.1 percent decline in physician offices ... From 2009 to 2013, the volume of E/M office visits provided to Medicare beneficiaries in HOPDs increased at an average annual rate of 9.2 percent, from 20.3 million visits to 28.9 million visits."

—Medicare Payment Policy – *Report to the Congress*, 2015.

The government has been studying the increase in provider-based clinics for many years and has noted that hospitals are acquiring these clinics for various reasons. The OIG noted in 1999 that "[f]or hospitals, one of the major reasons to purchase physician practices is to establish physician networks to compete with managed care products being offered by insurance companies" (HHS OIG, Hospital Ownership of Physician Practices, OEI-05-98-00110, 1999). Other studies show that hospitals are increasingly employing physicians in order to gain market share, "typically through lucrative service-line strategies," and to prepare "for expected Medicare reforms, including bundled payments, accountable care organizations (ACOs) and penalties for hospital readmissions" (Rising Hospital Employment of Physicians, 2011). Physicians reportedly are seeking integration with hospitals due to "stagnant reimbursement rates in the face of rising costs of private practice and a desire for better work-life balance" (Rising Hospital Employment of Physicians, 2011). MedPac has also theorized that hospitals and physicians may be incentivized to operate provider-based clinics simply to increase payment for outpatient services (Medicare Payment Policy – *Report to the Congress*, 2015).

Anecdotally, it appears that hospitals may acquire or open provider-based clinics to ensure that certain medical services are consistently available for the patient population in the surrounding community. This is especially true in rural areas where it is difficult to attract medical specialists who are likely to garner more income in urban areas. Teaching hospitals connected with universities may also wish to be able to offer a wide range of specialty outpatient medical services, to promote the hospital's public visibility and brand name and to promote research in specific medical areas by attracting top medical researchers. Hospitals may also be incentivized for other reasons; for example, the ability to count the medical residents in these departments in the hospital's indirect medical education (IME)/graduate medical education (GME) full-time equivalent (FTE) count, the use of these hospital-based physicians to count as participants for the CMS Electronic Health Record (EHR) Incentive Programs, and the ability for nonprofit hospitals to purchase drugs at discounted prices under the Public Health Service Act 340B discount drug program for these locations.

MedPac raised concerns about this shift in medical care to hospital outpatient departments because:

> "[A]mong other effects, the shift in care setting increases Medicare program spending and beneficiary cost-sharing liability because Medicare payment rates for the same or similar services are generally higher in HOPDs than in freestanding offices … As more E/M office visits are provided in HOPDs, the higher payment rates in the OPPS relative to the physician fee schedule result in increasingly higher program spending and beneficiary cost sharing. For example, we estimate that the Medicare program spent $1 billion more in 2009 and $1.5 billion more in 2013 than it would have if payment rates for E/M office visits were the same in HOPDs and freestanding offices. Analogously, beneficiaries' cost sharing was $260 million higher in 2009 and $370 million higher in 2013 than it would have been because of the higher rates paid in HOPD settings."

—Medicare Payment Policy – *Report to the Congress*, 2015.

With this increased rate of payment from Medicare, beneficiaries have also raised concerns about the increased patient financial liability for services furnished at provider-based departments. Most Medicare beneficiaries do not fully understand the reason for this increased cost, especially since provider-based clinics often appear to be nearly identical to freestanding physician offices, and there is no difference in the actual services received. In fact, beneficiaries have become increasingly vocal about the inequities they perceive in such a system. Therefore, MedPac, CMS, and OIG have been put under more and more pressure to both explain the higher payments for services furnished in provider-based clinics and ensure that the services are justifiable.

As a result, MedPac has for years recommended equalization of payments between physician office settings and hospital outpatient departments:

> "A greater concern is that the billing of many services has been migrating from physicians' offices to the usually higher-paid HOPD setting. This migration has resulted in higher spending for the Medicare program and higher cost sharing for Medicare beneficiaries without significant changes in patient care. Therefore, payment variations across ambulatory settings should be immediately addressed. Although it is reasonable to pay higher rates in HOPDs for certain services, we have developed criteria to identify services for which payment rates should be equal across settings or the differences should be narrowed. We encourage CMS to seek legislative authority to implement our recommendations to set equal payment rates for evaluation and management (E/M) office visits across settings and to align payment rates across settings for additional, select groups of services.
>
> To move toward paying equivalent rates for the same service across different sites of care, in 2014 we recommended adjusting the rates for certain services when they are provided in hospital outpatient departments (HOPDs) so they more closely align with the rates paid in freestanding physician offices."
>
> —Medicare Payment Policy – *Report to the Congress*, 2015.

MedPac gave some specific examples of the cost savings that would result from equalization of payment rates for the same services between freestanding and outpatient hospital departments:

> "For example, Medicare paid more than twice as much for a Level II echocardiogram in an outpatient facility ($492) as it did in a freestanding physician office ($228). This payment difference creates a financial incentive for hospitals to purchase freestanding physicians' offices and convert them to HOPDs without changing their location or patient mix. For example, if a hospital purchased a cardiologist's practice and redesignated that office as part of the hospital, the echocardiograms in that office would be billed as HOPD echocardiograms rather than physician-office echocardiograms, even if there were no change in the physician providing the service, the location of the physician's office, or the equipment being used. In 2013, the volume of echocardiograms billed as HOPD services increased 7 percent, while those billed [as] physician-office services declined 8 percent. This type of shift to the higher cost site of care increases program costs and costs for the beneficiary. The Commission's 2014 recommendation would reduce Medicare program spending, reduce beneficiary

*cost sharing, and create an incentive to improve efficiency by caring for patients in
the most efficient site for their condition."*

—Medicare Payment Policy – *Report to the Congress*, 2015.

Because of the increased overall cost for provider-based services and the pressure from the public, CMS and the OIG are increasing their scrutiny of the billing for these services. The OIG and
CMS have also openly begun to question the appropriateness of paying more for hospital-based
services overall and have begun to investigate whether these clinics are really incurring
increased costs as compared to independent physician offices.

Although CMS has resisted this pressure from MedPac so far, and continues to support the differential payment scheme, there are many signs that this criticism may lead to an eventual drop in
reimbursement for provider-based services, especially in off-campus provider-based departments
that are so similar to freestanding physician offices. CMS has also put in place a stricter regulatory structure around provider-based entities, especially off-campus departments. These regulations help ensure that these entities are truly operated as hospital facilities and not as independent clinics in disguise that are inappropriately billing under the hospital to receive the higher
provider-based payment. Because the off-campus locations are more prone to problems, the criteria are even stricter for those entities. In addition, CMS and the OIG are increasingly enforcing
these requirements.

With the new -PO modifier required for provider-based billing in 2016 and the new POS code
required for professional billing for hospital outpatient services furnished in off-campus locations
in 2016, CMS will have all the information necessary to focus audits on hospitals and physicians
that are most likely to be billing in error. In addition, analysis of this data may lead to future
reduction in payments, especially for off-campus provider-based departments. MedPac applauds
the use of these new tools:

> *"The proposal to collect data on services provided in off-campus provider-based
> departments through the claims process may have some value in helping policy-
> makers understand the growing trend of hospitals acquiring physician practices.
> The information may also help CMS verify that PFS [physician fee schedule] claims
> include the correct site of service. However, the proposal does not address the fun-
> damental problem of unjustified payment differences between settings. The PFS
> payment rate is usually higher when a service is provided in a nonfacility setting
> (such as a freestanding office) than a facility setting (such as an HOPD). PFS claims
> for services furnished in provider-based departments should indicate that the service
> was provided in a facility and should therefore receive the lower facility amount.
> However, there may be cases where the claim incorrectly indicates that the service*

was provided in a nonfacility setting. If this occurs, CMS could use the proposed modifier to check whether the service was furnished in a provider-based department and pay the appropriate rate."

—MedPAC comment, 2014.

So What Now?

You have already taken the first step. The fact that you are reading this means that you have identified that you do not have all of the information you need to know about provider-based entities, and you are ready to learn more and take on the task of assisting the hospital in auditing for compliance with these requirements. Now read on ... you will soon gain expertise in provider-based billing and auditing for compliance in this area.

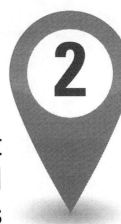

Departments and Entities Not Subject to Provider-Based Requirements

Hospital Departments *Not* Subject to Provider-Based Criteria

Before we further discuss the requirements to be a provider-based department, it is helpful to detail the types of hospital departments that do *not* have to be scrutinized under the provider-based criteria. According to the regulations governing provider-based facilities (42 *CFR* §413.65, 2011), there are four types of departments, units, entities, or facilities that a hospital does not need to include in its review of provider-based criteria, regardless of the location of these units on or off the hospital campus:

- Units that do not furnish billable clinical services

- Units, departments, and entities owned and operated by the hospital but separately certified

- Freestanding facilities

- Services furnished by another entity "under arrangements"

Units That Do *Not* Furnish Billable Clinical Services

A hospital unit must provide billable clinical services in order to be considered a provider-based department. Therefore, administrative departments or units of the hospital that do not furnish billable clinical services are not considered to be provider-based departments. These include, for example:

- Laundry

- Medical records

- Materials management

- Compliance

- Nursing administration

- Volunteers

- Biomedical engineering

- Patient financial services

- Public relations

- Central supply

- Transport services

- Utilization management

- Performance improvement

- Dietary

- Admitting

- Security

- Pharmacy

These departments all interface with patients and families daily and furnish essential hospital functions and certain types of essential services to the patients (e.g., food services, sterile equipment, transportation to diagnostic services, security, medications). In addition, these services are all subject to various state licensing, CMS certification, and/or accreditation requirements. However, these departments either do not furnish clinical services, or the clinical services they furnish are not separately billable to third-party payers, including Medicare. Therefore, the CMS provider-based regulations do not apply to these departments.

© 2015 HCPro

Clinical Units, Departments, and Entities Owned and Operated by the Hospital, but Billed Separately From the Hospital's Medicare Provider Number

Some entities and units owned and operated by a hospital are certified by Medicare under a provider or supplier number that is separate and distinct from the hospital's provider number and, therefore, are not subject to the provider-based requirements. These entities include the following types of Medicare providers and suppliers (42 *CFR* §413.65[a][ii], 2011):

- **Ambulatory surgery centers (ASC) that have a separate Medicare supplier number.**

  "An ASC is a distinct entity that operates exclusively for the purpose of furnishing outpatient surgical services to patients. It enters into an agreement with CMS to do so. An ASC is either independent (i.e., not a part of a provider of services or any other facility), or operated by a hospital (i.e., under the common ownership, licensure, or control of a hospital)."

  —*Medicare General Information and Eligibility Manual*, Chapter 5, §90.1

  ASCs furnish these surgical services to patients who do not require inpatient hospitalization and whose expected duration of services would not exceed 24 hours (42 *CFR* §416.2, 2010). ASCs must meet the Conditions of Coverage (CoCs) found in 42 *CFR* §§416.40–416.49 (2012).

  ASCs that are under the common ownership, licensure, or control of a hospital must:

  - "Elect to be separately certified as an ASC

  - Be a separately identifiable entity that is physically, administratively, and financially independent and distinct from other operations of the hospital with costs for the ASC treated as a non-reimbursable cost center on the hospital's cost report

  - Meet all the requirements with regard to health and safety, and agree to the assignment, coverage, and payment rules applied to independent ASCs

  - Be surveyed and approved as complying with the conditions for coverage for ASCs in 42 *CFR* 416.25-49."

  —*Medicare Claims Processing Manual*, Chapter 14, §10.1, 2014.

ASCs are reimbursed under a special ASC fee schedule (42 *CFR* §§416.120-160). Separately certified ASCs are different from hospital outpatient departments that may also furnish surgical services but are not separately certified. Hospitals may refer to these as outpatient surgery centers, or even ambulatory surgical centers. Therefore, it is essential that auditors ascertain whether this location has been issued a separate Medicare certification as an ASC before deciding whether this location must be audited as a provider-based location.

- **Comprehensive outpatient rehabilitation facilities (CORF).** A CORF is a nonresidential facility that is established and operated exclusively for the purpose of providing diagnostic, therapeutic, and restorative services to outpatients for the rehabilitation of injured, disabled, or sick persons at a single fixed location by or under the supervision of a physician (42 *CFR* §485.51, 2011). A CORF must be certified by CMS and meet the certification requirements listed in 42 *CFR* §§485.50–485.74 (2011). CORFs are reimbursed under the MPFS and subject to the same limitations described below for therapy services (*Medicare Claims Processing Manual*, Chapter 5, §§10–10.1, 2015). As is the case with ASCs, there is often confusion between CORFs and regular outpatient hospital therapy departments. The distinction between the two is whether or not the location has been separately certified by Medicare as a CORF.

- **HHAs** furnish skilled nursing, therapy, and other services to homebound patients in their place of residence (*Medicare Benefit Policy Manual*, Chapter 7, 2015). An HHA must meet the *Conditions of Participation* (*CoPs*) found in 42 *CFR* Part 484 in order to be reimbursed for these services (42 *CFR* §409.41, 2011). For example, under 42 *CFR* §484.14 (2011), the HHA is required to have its own governing body and administrator, among other things. CMS also mandates that HHAs establish a plan of care for each of its patients (42 *CFR* §484.18, 2007), must establish a group of professional personnel that oversees the HHA's clinical operations (42 *CFR* §484.16, 2011), must maintain a clinical record for each patient (42 *CFR* §484.48, 2011), and must furnish specific clinical services in accordance with the regulations (42 *CFR* §§484.30–38, 2011).

- **SNFs.** A SNF is defined in §1819(a) of the Social Security Act (n. d.) and 42 *CFR* 488.301 (2011) as a facility that:

  - Is primarily engaged in providing skilled nursing care and related services to residents who require medical or nursing care, or is primarily engaged in providing skilled rehabilitation services for the rehabilitation of injured, disabled, or sick residents and is not primarily for the care and treatment of mental diseases

  - Has in effect a transfer agreement with one or more Medicare participating hospitals

- Meets the requirements for a skilled nursing facility (SNF) described in 42 *CFR* 483, Subpart B (2011)

SNFs are reimbursed under a SNF PPS (42 *CFR* Part 413, Subpart J, 2011). Hospitals may operate a SNF as a "distinct part" of the hospital (referred to as distinct part SNFs). CMS specifically stated that distinct part SNFs must meet requirements other than the provider-based rules.

"The distinct part certification requirements set forth in §483.5 are separate and apart from the requirements to be considered "provider based" as set forth in §413.65. Indeed, SNFs are no longer required to request or be approved for provider-based status and are not subject to the provider based regulations in §413.65. Moreover, simply meeting the provider-based requirements, which, as we have previously stated do not apply to SNFs, does not translate to automatically meeting the distinct part requirements. Accordingly, we will evaluate each request for approval of a distinct part SNF or NF against the criteria outlined in §483.5."

—68 *Fed. Reg.* 46036, 46063, 2003.

- **Hospices** furnish "a comprehensive set of services described in §1861(dd)(1) of the Social Security Act (n. d.), identified and coordinated by an interdisciplinary group to provide for the physical, psychosocial, spiritual, and emotional needs of a terminally ill patient and/or family members, as delineated in a specific patient plan of care" (42 *CFR* §418.3, 2014). CMS must certify hospices to provide hospice care (42 *CFR* Part 418, Subpart C, 2011). Hospices are reimbursed a per diem amount for different levels of hospice care—routine, general inpatient, continuous care, and respite care (42 *CFR* Part 418, Subpart G, 2011).

- **Inpatient rehabilitation units (IRF).** An IRF is a hospital or hospital unit that has been excluded from the hospital inpatient PPS (IPPS) and serves an inpatient population of whom a specified percent require intensive rehabilitation services (42 *CFR* 412.622[a][3], 2011). IRFs must meet the *CoP*s found in 42 *CFR* §412.604. IRFs are made under a separate IRF PPS.

- **Durable medical equipment, prosthetic, and orthotic (DMEPOS).** DMEPOS suppliers are certified by Medicare to sell or rent Medicare-covered DMEPOS (42 *CFR* §424.57, 2014). DMEPOS suppliers must meet specific conditions of payment (42 *CFR* §424.57[b], 2014). These services are reimbursed under a special set of DMEPOS fee schedules (42 *CFR* §414.210, 2011). Finally, these services are billed to and paid by the Durable Medical Equipment MAC (DME MAC) assigned to the DMEPOS service area, rather than the hospital's Part A/Part B MAC.

- **Dialysis facilities.** A dialysis facility is an entity that provides outpatient maintenance dialysis services, home dialysis training and support services, or both. "A dialysis facility may be an independent or hospital-based unit ... [including] a self-care dialysis unit that furnishes only self-dialysis services" (42 *CFR* §494.10, 2011).

- **Independent diagnostic testing facilities (IDTF).** An IDTF is an entity that furnishes diagnostic services such as magnetic resonance imaging (MRI), computed tomography scans (CT), and other radiology and diagnostic services. An IDTF is independent of hospitals and physician offices but is paid under the MPFS (42 *CFR* §410.33, 2011). IDTFs must meet the Medicare conditions listed in 42 *CFR* §410.33(g) (2011).

  Most hospitals offer the same diagnostic services as IDTFs (e.g., MRI, CT, radiology) but do not have these services certified as a freestanding IDTF. Therefore, auditors should ensure that the diagnostic center is certified by Medicare as an IDTF prior to excluding the location from review under the provider-based requirements.

- **Physical therapy (PT), occupational therapy (OT), and speech-language pathology (SLP) therapy facilities.** PT, OT, and SLP therapy facilities furnish only covered PT, OT, and/or SLP services to ambulatory patients *outside of* hospitals and critical access hospitals (CAH). These facilities bill Medicare independently for the services provided (42 *CFR* §§410.59, 410.60, and 410.62, 2011). There is an annual financial cap on the amount of payment for these services (42 *CFR* §410.60(e), 2011).

- **Ambulances.** Ambulance services are covered as defined in 42 *CFR* §410.40 (2010). For example, the following types of medically necessary ambulance services are covered for Medicare beneficiaries who are not able to ambulate, are unable to get up from bed without assistance, and are unable to sit in a chair or wheelchair:

  - Basic life support (emergency and nonemergency)

  - Advanced life support (ALS), level 1 (emergency and nonemergency)

  - ALS, level 2

  - Paramedic ALS intercept

  - Specialty care transport

  - Fixed wing transport

  - Rotary wing transport

  Medicare also covers nonemergency, scheduled, repetitive ambulance services if ordered by the patient's physician with a certification that the patient meets the conditions listed above.

 © 2015 HCPro

Ambulance suppliers must meet the requirements detailed in 42 *CFR* §410.41 (2011). Specifically, CMS lays out criteria for the ambulance vehicle, staffing, and billing that must be met in order for an ambulance company to be certified to furnish and bill for ambulance services. The ambulance company must complete and submit an application to the MAC to be certified as an ambulance supplier.

- **Rural health clinics (RHC) affiliated with hospitals having 50 or more beds.** RHCs are covered by Medicare to furnish Part B services in medically underserved areas (42 *CFR* §§405.2411–405.2417, 2011). An RHC must be certified by CMS to bill for these covered services (42 *CFR* §405.2402, 2011). RHCs are paid for these services on a reasonable cost basis if they are operated under the ownership and control of a hospital, SNF, or HHA. If the RHC is an independent facility, it receives an all-inclusive rate per beneficiary visit (42 *CFR* §405.2462, 2006).

  Notably, because these facilities are all certified independently from the hospital, none of these types of entities are subject to the three-day payment window (see Chapter 5).

Because these entities are separately certified, they are required to comply with the specific *CoPs* or *CoCs* applicable to these types of providers or suppliers. In addition, these entities are required to submit claims to CMS under their own provider/supplier number, rather than with the hospital Medicare number and name. Therefore, they receive payment for their own services separate from the hospital. The reimbursement for these separately certified entities is calculated based on Medicare payment schemes that are separate and different from the hospital IPPS or outpatient prospective payment system (OPPS). Finally, CMS may require these entities to submit Medicare cost reports separate from the hospital. At a minimum, CMS may require the hospital to separate the costs for these entities from its own costs on the Medicare cost report.

While these separately certified entities may be owned by the corporation that also operates the hospital, they are not really part of hospital operations in terms of being certified and regulated by CMS. Because these entities are separately certified, they are governed by their own distinct set of *CoPs* or *CoCs* and, therefore, are not subject to the hospital *CoPs*, are not considered to be provider-based departments, and are not subject to the provider-based criteria (42 *CFR* §413.65[a][ii], 2011). This is true even if the unit or department is listed on the hospital's state license.

Freestanding Facilities or Entities

Hospitals frequently have close relationships with freestanding facilities that furnish services that are separate from the hospital license and Medicare certification, are not billed by the hospital to third-party payers, and are not accounted for on the hospital's cost report. These are distinct from the separately certified providers and suppliers listed above that are actually owned and operated by the hospital and may even be included on the hospital license. The relationship freestanding entities have with the hospital generally falls into one of the two following categories defined by the ownership and operation of the facility:

- **Entities not owned or operated by the hospital.** Historically, hospitals lease space on campus and in hospital-owned buildings to healthcare providers and entities that are owned and operated by a corporation that is completely separate from the hospital. The hospital generally has absolutely no investment or legal interest in these companies. These healthcare providers may be important to the hospital's strategic goals and patient referral base, which may prompt the hospital to create these relationships. However, under the CMS regulations, these entities are not provider-based departments and are not subject to the provider-based rules.

  For example, physician offices owned and operated by medical groups frequently lease space in hospital-owned medical office buildings. In fact, many hospitals may actually lease office space within the four walls of the main hospital building to these physicians. These physicians often have medical staff privileges at the hospital, and patients are followed by these physicians in their clinics before and after inpatient hospitalizations. In addition, the hospital usually has a close and important relationship with these physicians, who are often responsible for the majority of the medical and surgical care furnished at the hospital. Finally, these physicians are instrumental in formulating standards of medical care at the hospital through the hospital's organized medical staff and committees.

  However, since these clinics are not owned by the hospital, the services furnished in these locations are not billed under the hospital's name or provider number. Therefore, these clinics are not considered to be provider-based departments of the hospital and are not subject to the provider-based rules. Instead, the services are billed under the name and Medicare numbers of the physician or medical group on a CMS 1500 (837P electronic form) with POS code 11.

  Similarly, other types of providers and suppliers (e.g., HHAs, laboratories, hospices, SNFs, dialysis units, other unrelated hospitals) owned by other companies may lease space on the hospital campus without being owned or operated by the hospital. The services furnished by these entities generally complement those of the hospital, which may refer patients to these entities or vice versa. However, since these entities are not owned by the hospital, the services furnished in these locations are not billed under the hospital's name or provider number. Therefore, they are not considered to be provider-based departments of the hospital and are not subject to the provider-based rules. Instead, these services are billed under the name and Medicare numbers of the separately owned entities. These entities would not be included in the hospital's cost report.

 © 2015 HCPro

Notably, none of these types of entities are subject to the three-day payment window discussed in Chapter 5, because they are not part of the hospital.

- **Entities owned but not operated by the hospital.** As discussed in Chapter 1, hospitals generally are incentivized to operate provider-based clinics to ensure that certain medical services are consistently available for the patient population, to promote the hospital's public visibility and brand name, to promote research in specific medical areas, and possibly to increase payment for outpatient services.

  If the corporation operating a hospital recognizes that there is a shortage of specialists in an area, it may be compelled to find a way to financially support their continued presence so the hospital's patients may benefit from the services furnished by these specialists. However, if the hospital cannot or does not want to integrate these clinics as provider-based departments, or otherwise understands that the specialists would not want to give up overall control to the hospital, the entity may become a freestanding clinic that is owned but not operated by the hospital. This type of arrangement often occurs with CAHs in rural medical shortage areas. It is frequently difficult to incentivize medical specialists to remain in rural areas, and the financial support offered by the CAH to the facility tips the balance to keep these essential services in the area.

  In these cases, even though the hospital invests in and legally owns these freestanding physician offices/clinics, a decision has been made that the hospital will not operate the clinics as provider-based departments. Instead, the clinics continue to operate as freestanding clinics under the day-to-day operational control of the physician/medical group and are billed under the name and Medicare numbers of the physician or medical group on a CMS-1500 claim form (837P electronic form) with POS code 11. The services furnished in these locations are not billed under the hospital's name or provider number. Therefore, the clinics are not considered to be provider-based departments of the hospital and are not subject to the provider-based rules.

  Interestingly, these hospital-owned freestanding clinics are subject to certain aspects of the three-day payment window discussed in Chapter 5.

The freestanding facility should take all the necessary steps to maintain its independent status and should not give the impression that it is a provider-based department. The hospital must ensure that there is no signage at the freestanding facility that identifies it as a hospital department—it is best if the hospital name does not appear on the sign for the freestanding facility.

With regard to freestanding clinics, the hospital should also:

- Audit the cost report to ensure the space is carved out of the statistics, costs, and expenses included on the cost report

- Ensure the patients seen in the freestanding facility are not registered as hospital outpatients

- Ensure the hospital is not billing for the facility services furnished at the freestanding facility. The services furnished at the freestanding physician office should be billed on a CMS 1500 (837P electronic form) with POS code 11, rather than with POS code 22. Billing must be done under the name and numerical identifiers of the physician or medical group that operates the office/clinic.

The hospital should audit to ensure that there is a formal contract in place between the hospital and the freestanding facility, and that the contract between the hospital and freestanding facility is based on a fair market valuation. It is recommended that a qualified legal review be undertaken to verify that the relationship between the parties meets all applicable legal requirements and that the freestanding facility could not be mistaken for a provider-based department.

Services Furnished to Hospital Patients by Other Entities "Under Arrangements"

Hospitals are required to furnish all covered services to Medicare beneficiaries who are inpatients or outpatients either directly or "under arrangements" (42 *CFR* 412.50[c], 2011). A hospital may not always be able to furnish every type of service required by patients through its own employees and on its own hospital campus. For this reason, hospitals often enter into contractual arrangements with other entities to provide services using the employees of another entity rather than the hospital's employees. At times, these services are furnished on the hospital premises. However, many times they are furnished in remote offices owned and operated by the other entity. Whether performed on or off the hospital campus, these are referred to as services furnished "under arrangements" (*see* 42 *USC* §1395x[w], 2011; 42 *USC* §1395x[b][3], 2011; 42 *CFR* §409.3, 2011; *General Information and Eligibility Manual,* Chapter 5, §10.3, 2009).

For example, a hospital may decide to contract with a freestanding radiology company or IDTF to furnish MRI services under arrangements for its hospital patients. This may be a more economical approach than if a hospital operates its own MRI with full-time hospital employees. It is also an option if the open MRI operated by the IDTF is only rarely required by the hospital patients. The entity that furnishes these services is not owned or operated by the hospital, but instead has a contractual arrangement whereby the outside entity furnishes a specific volume of services at defined rates, and the hospital maintains a certain level of oversight and control over these services.

Medicare payment regulations and some state licensing requirements place limitations on the types of services that may be furnished under arrangements. The goal of these limitations is to ensure that the hospital is not just serving as a shell billing agent or mechanism for the other party and is actually functioning as the provider of hospital services. CMS has stated that a hospital may only furnish services under arrangements that are "specialized healthcare services that it does not itself offer and that are needed to supplement the range of services that the provider does offer its patients" (67 *Fed. Reg.* 49982, 50091, 2002). CMS noted that it intends to ensure that most of the hospital services are furnished by the hospital through its own employees and prevent the wholesale exportation of clinical hospital services:

> "It is possible that all or virtually all services needed to operate a facility could be obtained under contract, resulting in nothing more than a nominal connection between the facility and the provider that claims it as an integral and subordinate part. To prevent a facility operated in this way from inappropriately claiming to be part of a provider, reasonable controls on management contracts are needed."

> —67 *Fed. Reg.* 49982, 50091, 2002.

CMS promulgated a final rule that would not allow hospitals to furnish routine services like dietary, room and board, and nursing services under arrangements outside of the hospital, although the effective date of this rule was extended several times to January 1, 2015.

> "Because there are hospitals in the midst of significant building projects that, when completed, will enable the hospital to provide routine services in compliance with the requirements of this revised policy, we believe it is appropriate to further delay the effective date. We stated that we expect that, with the additional time before the revised 'under arrangement' policy becomes effective, hospitals will complete the work needed to ensure compliance with the new requirement. Effective for services provided on or after January 1, 2015, all hospitals would need to be in full compliance with the revised policy for services furnished under arrangement."

> —78 *Fed. Reg.* 50496, 50744, 2013.

The result of this rule is that effective January 1, 2015, the only services that may be furnished by hospitals under arrangements are diagnostic services like CTs and MRIs.

Certain cancer hospitals continue to oppose the enforcement of this requirement, but CMS stated that the "virtual discharge" arrangement proposed would violate the hospital *CoPs*.

> "PPS-excluded cancer hospitals that are co-located with IPPS hospitals are most affected by the proposed policy and, along with the alliance representing these hospitals, made further comments that repeated their objections to this policy raised in last year's rule. These commenters expressed concern that it could compromise

patient care, that the policy is a reversal of CMS' guidance the hospitals received while each hospital was seeking co-located status … . They believed that their proposal would allow the hospital to continue moving patients to its host hospital for particular services, without discharging the patient, as is currently done. The commenters added that after the patient is formally discharged, each hospital would separately bill Medicare for the services it provided the discharged patient.

The 'virtual discharge' proposal … is unacceptable from a CoP perspective because the co-located hospital and the cancer hospital are two separately certified hospitals for purposes of Medicare participation. Therefore, moving the patient from the cancer hospital to the co-located IPPS hospital would require the patient to be discharged."

—78 Fed. Reg. 50496, 50744-45, 2013.

CMS requires that the entity that furnishes the services under arrangements bill the hospital rather than billing the Medicare beneficiary or the Medicare program for these services. As a result, payment by the hospital must discharge the liability of the beneficiary or any other party to pay for the items or services (42 *CFR* 409.3, 1996). In other words, the entity that furnishes services under arrangements must accept the contracted amount as payment in full for the services, and may not bill anyone else for the excess charge not reimbursed by the hospital.

Certain state licensing laws may also limit the types of services that may be furnished under arrangements.

Under the Medicare payment rules and *CoPs*, CMS requires that the hospital exercise a certain amount of professional oversight and control over the services furnished by other entities under arrangements. The *General Information and Eligibility Manual* states that:

"A provider may have others furnish certain covered items and services to their patients through arrangements under which receipt of payment by the provider for the services discharges the liability of the beneficiary or any other person to pay for the service. In permitting providers to furnish services under arrangements, it was not intended that the provider merely serve as a billing mechanism for the other party. Accordingly, for services provided under arrangements to be covered, the provider must exercise professional responsibility over the arranged-for services. The provider's professional supervision over arranged-for services requires application of many of the same quality controls as are applied to services furnished by salaried employees. The provider must accept the patient for treatment in accordance with its admission policies, and maintain a complete and timely clinical record on the

patient, which includes diagnoses, medical history, physician's orders, and progress notes relating to all services received, and must maintain liaison with the attending physician regarding the progress of the patient and the need for revised orders."

—*General Information and Eligibility Manual,* Chapter 5, §10.3, 2009.

The hospital *CoPs* state that:

"The governing body must be responsible for services furnished in the hospital whether or not they are furnished under contracts. The governing body must ensure that a contractor of services (including one for shared services and joint ventures) furnishes services that permit the hospital to comply with all applicable conditions of participation and standards for the contracted services.

(1) The governing body must ensure that the services performed under a contract are provided in a safe and effective manner.

(2) The hospital must maintain a list of all contracted services, including the scope and nature of the services provided."

—*42 CFR* §482.12(e), 2011.

Because the hospital is already required to oversee the services furnished by a contractor under arrangements in accordance with the regulations cited above, CMS does not require that the hospital also meet the provider-based requirements for these services. In essence, applying the provider-based requirements to these departments would be duplicative of the regulations governing services furnished under arrangements.

Scenarios

The following scenarios will assist in providing a more complete understanding of the circumstances where the provider-based requirements do not apply.

Scenario A

ABC Hospital is located in a rural location where it is difficult to find specialty physicians to provide services to its hospital outpatients. The following facilities furnish services on or near the hospital campus:

- A Medicare-certified HHA owned by the hospital. The HHA staff are employed by the hospital.

- Internal medicine, surgery, and pediatric clinics operated by the hospital in a hospital-owned building on the main hospital campus. The clinics are staffed by hospital employees, and the patients treated in the clinics are registered and billed as hospital outpatients.

- A nephrology clinic located five miles from the hospital campus that is owned by the hospital. The hospital purchased the location to ensure that the nephrology services are available in the community but agreed to allow the nephrology group to continue to operate the location. The patients treated in the off-campus nephrology clinic are registered and billed as physician office patients. The nephrologists from the off-campus nephrology clinic have hospital medical staff privileges and consult on patients seen in the internal medicine clinic, as necessary.

The hospital compliance officer has asked you to list the departments that are excluded from the provider-based requirements. You explain to the compliance officer that the following are excluded from the provider-based requirements, based on the reasons stated:

- The hospital-owned and operated HHA. The HHA is separately certified by Medicare and, therefore, the patients treated by the HHA are admitted to the HHA and billed separately as HHA patients under the name and provider number of the HHA. The HHA must meet the HHA *CoPs*. Therefore, this separately certified entity is not subject to the provider-based requirements.

- The off-campus hospital-owned nephrology clinic. Even though it is owned by the hospital, it is operated as a freestanding physician office clinic. Therefore, it is not a provider-based department.

Scenario B

After you finish the exhausting job of auditing the hospital's provider-based clinics and turn in your report, the CEO calls you in and demands to know why you didn't audit the following locations:

- A laboratory operated by another corporation that is leasing space in the hospital-owned medical office building. Patients who receive services in the laboratory are not registered as hospital outpatients.

- A PT department operated in a hospital-owned building attached to the main hospital building. The hospital has a contract with "Magic Hands PT Group" to manage and furnish employees for the PT department. The patients receiving services in the PT department are registered as hospital outpatients.

- A peritoneal dialysis unit owned and operated by the hospital, located in a hospital-owned building immediately adjacent to the main hospital building and staffed by hospital employees.

- The hospital infection control offices located in the basement of a hospital-owned medical office building a block from the hospital. Infection control activities for hospital inpatients and outpatients are required by the Medicare *CoPs* and state licensing laws.

You explain that all of these locations are excluded from the provider-based requirements, as follows:

- The laboratory is owned and operated by another corporation, and is not a hospital outpatient department, even though it is operated in a hospital-owned space. Therefore, this freestanding entity is not subject to the hospital provider-based requirements.

- The PT department furnishes services to hospital outpatients "under arrangements." The hospital is required to oversee these services under different regulations, but it is not required to ensure that the location also meets the provider-based requirements.

- The peritoneal dialysis unit is separately certified by Medicare. While it must comply with the Medicare dialysis facility requirements, it is not required to meet the provider-based requirements.

- The hospital infection control offices are administrative services. While these services are required by the Medicare CoPs and state licensing requirements, they are not clinical services that are separately billed to Medicare or any other third-party payer. Therefore, the provider-based requirements do not apply to these services.

Scenario C

You have called the hospital managers together to begin your audit of provider-based departments. The managers of the following two services claim that these services are excluded from the provider-based requirements:

- A hospital outpatient surgical clinic staffed by hospital employees. The department is commonly referred to by the staff as an ambulatory surgery center (ASC). However, the clinic is not certified by Medicare as an ASC.

- A phlebotomy station owned by the hospital located in a space leased by the hospital in a nearby retail space owned by another business. It is staffed by hospital employees and the patients seen in the phlebotomy station are registered as hospital outpatients.

You explain that these areas are subject to the provider-based requirements, as follows:

- The hospital outpatient surgical clinic is not separately certified by Medicare as an ASC. Therefore, the patients that are treated there are registered and billed as hospital outpatients, rather than ASC patients, and these areas are required to meet the provider-based criteria.

- The phlebotomy station is an off-campus hospital outpatient department since the hospital owns and operates the services at that location, the services are furnished by hospital employees, and the patients are registered and billed as hospital outpatients. Therefore, the location is subject to the provider-based rules.

How to Qualify as a Provider-Based Department

3

Meeting Provider-Based Criteria

L ooking back at the prior chapter, we clarified that a hospital needs to be concerned about meeting provider-based criteria only for clinical departments that it determines fall under the hospital's license and Medicare certification and accreditation. Specifically, a hospital needs to be concerned about any department that furnishes clinical services that are billed under the hospital's name and Medicare provider number regardless of location in the hospital and whether it is on or off the hospital campus, unless those services are furnished under arrangements by another entity.

Type and Location of Provider-Based Departments

Before we discuss further the specific criteria that must be met to qualify as a provider-based department, understand that these requirements vary somewhat based on the location and type of provider-based department. There are four main types of provider-based departments to be concerned with that will be further discussed in this chapter:

- On-campus provider-based departments
- Off-campus provider-based departments
- Remote hospital locations
- Satellite hospital facilities

On-campus provider-based department

CMS has defined a hospital campus as the "physical area immediately adjacent to" the hospital's main buildings and other areas and structures that are within 250 yards of the main hospital that are not strictly contiguous to the main buildings (42 *CFR* §413.65[a][2], 2011). This sounds fairly straightforward. However, CMS has not clearly defined what it means by the "main hospital." Historically, hospitals have had fairly simple configurations, contained in only one large, square building. In those cases, it is fairly simple to determine the location of the main hospital and, hence, what is located more than 250 yards from the main hospital building. However, most modern hospitals have built adjacent buildings and structures to house outpatient and inpatient services and may even lease space from other companies to add to the hospital footprint. It is conceivable that a hospital campus could extend for many city blocks or miles as the hospital gradually expands and adds another building next to the previous ones. This is especially true in states like California that have enforced new earthquake building codes for hospitals, which caused most hospitals in that state to purchase adjacent land in order to build upgraded facilities.

The issue of clearly defining a hospital campus was raised in the public comments to the regulations, and CMS expressed at that time that this is a flexible definition, subject to discretion by CMS' Regional Offices (RO).

> *"This definition would encompass not only institutions that are located in self-contained, well-defined settings, but other locations, such as in central city areas, where there may be a group of buildings that function as a campus but are not strictly contiguous and may even be crossed by public streets. This would also allow the regional offices to determine, on a case-by-case basis, what comprises a hospital's campus. We believe allowing regional office discretion to make these determinations will allow us to take a flexible and realistic approach to the many physical configurations that hospitals and other providers can adopt."*

—65 *Fed. Reg.* 18434, 18511, 2000.

The ROs have the discretion to make a determination that a department located farther than 250 yards from the main hospital building is on-campus, but the hospital can also challenge this determination (In the Case of St. Vincent's Catholic Medical Centers of New York, *DAB Decision No. CR1734*, 2008). In 2008, CMS denied a request made by St. Vincent's Catholic Medical Centers of New York to designate a cancer center as an on-campus provider-based department because it was located 327 yards away from what CMS designated as the main hospital buildings—77 yards more than CMS allows for on-campus provider-based clinics. CMS also noted as negative factors: the dense urban nature of the location; lack of a direct line of sight between the hospital and the cancer center; travel from one facility to the other requiring a walk of more than 400 yards across three busy streets and a major avenue; and the presence of other businesses, residences, and activities between the facilities (In the Case of St. Vincent's, 2008). The Administrative Law Judge (ALJ) remanded the determination to CMS to reconsider the decision, noting that:

> "The Federal Register states that the definition of 'campus' encompasses 'not only institutions that are located in self-contained, well-defined settings, but other locations, such as in central city areas, where there may be a group of buildings that functions as a campus but are not strictly contiguous, and may even be crossed by public streets'. 65 Fed. Reg. 18434, 18511 (April 7, 2000). The Federal Register notes that such a definition gives the regional office discretion to make determinations, on a case-by-case basis, as to what constitutes a hospital's campus."

> —In the Case of St. Vincent's, 2008.

After stating that "off-campus facilities are subject to additional administrative requirements and restrictions (which can inhibit a main provider's ability to operate its facility efficiently), not imposed upon on-campus facilities," the ALJ noted that:

> "The determination whether to grant or deny an application for on-campus provider-based status must hinge on the objective to be achieved by the regulation, and the legitimate interests to be protected. Whether it is added beneficiary financial liability, quality of service, or personal safety, CMS must articulate, in precise terms, the basis for denial of a request for an on-campus provider-based determination."

> —In the Case of St. Vincent's, 2008.

The moral of this story is that hospitals should consider petitioning CMS for a determination that a provider-based department is on-campus, rather than off-campus, even if the department initially appears to be located more than 250 yards from some of the main hospital buildings. The key is to argue that the regulatory intent is met. In other words, the hospital may argue that its campus is larger than it appears at first glance and encompasses the provider-based department at issue, because the department does not require the additional scrutiny applicable to off-campus departments.

To accomplish this, the hospital should explain how the department is inextricably tied to the main hospital campus such that the additional criteria do not apply. This may involve demonstrating that the public views the department as an integral part of the main campus, that there is continuous traffic between the main hospital and the department, that the main hospital has such ties with the department that there is ongoing and immediate oversight over the services furnished there, and other similar factors. This may be worth the effort involved to avoid the additional administrative burden required for off-campus departments.

Off-campus provider-based department

As can be expected from its name, an off-campus department is any hospital department that is not determined to be an on-campus department (42 *CFR* §413.65[a][2], 2011). This means that generally the department is more than 250 yards from the hospital's main buildings, as well as the other main hospital areas and structures located within 250 yards of the main hospital (see Figure 3.1). However, in general, CMS does not expect that provider-based departments will be located more than 35 miles from the hospital campus, with some exceptions that demonstrate that the location outside of the 35-mile radius is integrated with the hospital despite the distance from the hospital (42 *CFR* §§413.65[a][3]–[e][3], 2011). This demonstrates that CMS does not generally expect that a hospital is typically capable of providing the proper oversight or management necessary for a provider-based department that is located more than 250 yards from the hospital. (Note that some state licensure laws also have definitions for on-campus and off-campus departments, but these requirements should not be confused with CMS' requirements.)

Figure 3.1	On-Campus and Off-Campus Provider-Based Departments

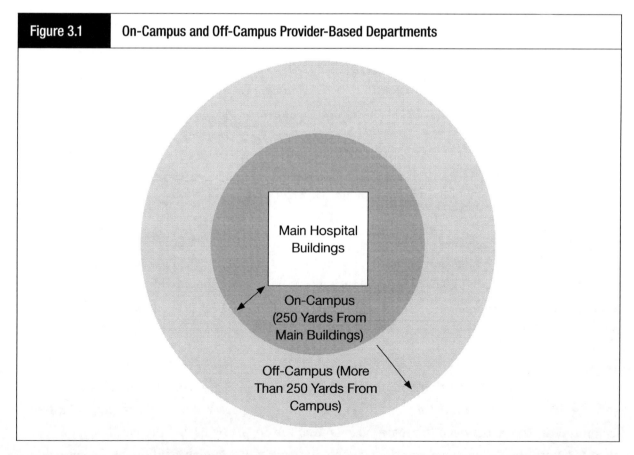

*Source: **Gina M. Reese, Esq., RN,** an instructor for HCPro's Medicare Boot Camp®—Hospital Version and Medicare Boot Camp®— Utilization Review Version. Reprinted with permission.*

 © 2015 HCPro

Remote location of a hospital

A remote location of a hospital is a "facility or organization that is either created or acquired by a hospital" for the "purpose of furnishing inpatient hospital services under the name, ownership and financial and administrative control of the main hospital" (42 *CFR* §413.65[a][2], 2011). A remote location of a hospital is not the same as a "satellite facility" as defined below. A hospital is operating a remote location when it opens another inpatient unit in a remote building (see Figure 3.2). The remote location is operated under the same Medicare and Medicaid provider numbers and state license as the main hospital.

If the services furnished at another location are operating under a different Medicare/Medicaid provider number or state license than the main hospital, this is not a remote location. Instead, that location is a separate hospital from the main hospital. The term "remote location" is never used to describe hospital *outpatient* services.

Figure 3.2	Remote Location of a Hospital

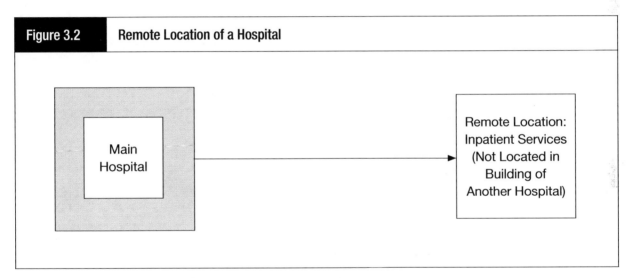

Source: **Gina M. Reese, Esq., RN,** *an instructor for HCPro's Medicare Boot Camp®—Hospital Version and Medicare Boot Camp®— Utilization Review Version. Reprinted with permission.*

Satellite hospital facility

A satellite facility is defined by CMS in 42 *CFR* §§412.22(h)(1) (2011) and 412.25(e)(1) (2010) as "part of a hospital that provides inpatient services in a building also used by another hospital, or in one or more entire buildings located on the same campus as buildings used by another hospital" (42 *CFR* §413.65[a][2], 2011).

Just like a remote location of a hospital, a satellite facility operates under the same Medicare/ Medicaid provider numbers and state license as the main hospital. If the services furnished at a so-called satellite facility are operating under a different Medicare/Medicaid provider number or state license, this is not actually a satellite facility. Instead, that location is a separate hospital from the main hospital.

The main difference between a remote location of a hospital and a satellite facility is that the latter is located and operated inside of another hospital (see Figure 3.3), whereas the former is operated in a location outside of another hospital. Notably, both remote locations and satellite facilities furnish inpatient, rather than outpatient, hospital services.

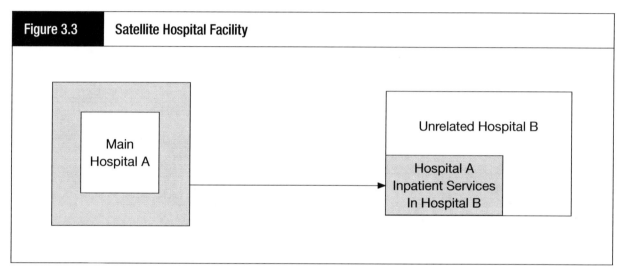

Figure 3.3   **Satellite Hospital Facility**

Main Hospital A

Unrelated Hospital B

Hospital A Inpatient Services In Hospital B

*Source: **Gina M. Reese, Esq., RN,** an instructor for HCPro's Medicare Boot Camp®—Hospital Version and Medicare Boot Camp®— Utilization Review Version. Reprinted with permission.*

Requirements to Qualify as a Provider-Based Entity

All of the provider-based requirements discussed boil down to one basic concept: The hospital must demonstrate that it treats each provider-based department as an integral part of the hospital. No provider-based department should be operated as if it is separate or distinct from the hospital. CMS articulated this succinctly in the *Federal Register*:

> *"The objective in issuing specific criteria for provider-based status is to ensure that higher levels of Medicare payment and increases in beneficiary liability for deductibles or coinsurance (which can all be associated with provider-based status) are limited to situations where the facility or organization is clearly and unequivocally an integral and subordinate part of a provider."*
>
> —65 *Fed. Reg.* 18434, 18506, 2000.

 © 2015 HCPro

The hospital need only remember this concept to resolve any questions that arise about how to comply with these requirements. If there are factors present that cause the public or the hospital to view the department as less integrated with the hospital than other hospital departments, there is a risk that this department is inappropriately being treated as provider-based.

It is not enough to just give this lip service, believe that it is true, or assume that it is sufficient to just slap the hospital's name on a clinic or department and hope that everyone will believe it is a hospital department. Instead, the hospital must ensure that there is no significant distinction between how it oversees and operates the provider-based department and any of its other hospital departments. All of the detailed CMS requirements listed below are designed to probe that basic requirement and ensure that the hospital has not allowed the department to operate outside of its control and oversight.

Threshold Requirements for All Provider-Based Departments

CMS outlined a number of basic requirements in 42 *CFR* §413.65 (2011) that apply to every provider-based department, regardless of whether it is located on or off the hospital campus (*Transmittal A-03-030*, 2003). These requirements also apply to remote locations of the hospital and satellite facilities, as defined above. The following is a discussion of these requirements.

Licensure

CMS requires that the main provider specifically request that the provider-based department, remote location, or satellite facility be added to or included in the hospital's state licensure. This means that the provider-based department is subject to state licensure surveys and requirements, including any life safety, earthquake, or other hospital requirements. The only exception to this requirement is when state law specifically prohibits the addition of the provider-based department, remote location, or satellite facility to the hospital license, or requires a separate license for the department, remote location, or satellite facility (42 *CFR* §413.65[d][1], 2011).

This criterion is generally easier to comply with if the hospital and hospital-based departments were constructed at the same time or under the same hospital planning scheme. The hospital is more likely to include provider-based departments on the application for state licensure if it is part of the original list of hospital departments. However, this may be more difficult to achieve if the hospital has recently absorbed or acquired locations that used to operate as freestanding physician clinics or other freestanding facilities, since these locations were not initially added to the hospital license and were likely built and operated under more lax standards. In addition, hospital leadership is more likely to neglect to add departments to the hospital license if they are added slowly over time, especially if there is no single person or department in charge of ensuring compliance with this requirement.

CMS denied provider-based status for an Oklahoma hospital in 2003 based on this licensure requirement. In that case, The Physicians' Hospital in Anadarko requested provider-based status for its rehabilitation services located in Chickasha, Oklahoma. However, CMS denied that request, because the rehabilitation services were not licensed by the state of Oklahoma, either separately or under the hospital license (The Physicians' Hospital In Anadarko, *DAB Decision No. CR1460*, 2006). In upholding that denial, the ALJ noted that Oklahoma law did not preclude the inclusion of the rehabilitation services under the hospital license.

The hospital argued on appeal that the services were eligible to be operated under the hospital license and that it had indeed requested that this location be included under the license, even though that request had not yet been granted. However, the Appellate Division of the Departmental Appeals Board (DAB) upheld the ALJ's denial of the provider-based status based on the hospital's failure to actually license the rehabilitation services under the hospital (The Physicians' Hospital In Anadarko, 2006).

It is not sufficient under this requirement, if a hospital has requested that the department be added to its license and that the department is being operated as a hospital department, if the state licensing agency has not yet actually approved that request. In Union Hospital, Inc., *DAB Decision No. CR2422* (2011), the hospital argued that it had requested that the State of Indiana add three clinics to its state license, and the American Osteopathic Association had "confirmed the operation of the three entities under standards deemed by CMS to verify compliance with the conditions of participation for hospitals." Union Hospital further argued that it operated the three clinics "in a manner that was indistinguishable from the way in which these entities would be operated, were they to be licensed in common" with the hospital (Union Hospital, Inc., 2011).

The ALJ upheld CMS' denial of provider-based status for these clinics, stating that:

> *"This argument fails as a matter of law. The regulation does not recognize an equivalent status to a common license. Thus, a facility does not establish itself to be a department of a hospital by proving that the manner in which it was operated was equivalent to being operated under the same license as the hospital. Nor may a facility argue that it met all the criteria for a common license but did not share a license for purely technical reasons. Finally, a facility may not argue that it should be 'deemed' to be licensed in common with a hospital because it met the standards of a private accreditation body."*

> —Union Hospital, Inc., 2011.

If the state where the hospital operates has a cost review commission or other such agency that "has the authority to regulate the rates charged by hospitals or other providers," it is important that the hospital obtain any rulings by that cost review commission regarding the provider-based department. If the cost control agency has ruled that the provider-based department is not part of the hospital, CMS will follow that ruling and also determine that the department is not provider-based (42 *CFR* §413.65[d][1], 2011).

At one time, state hospital rate-setting was in place in several states in an attempt to control hospital reimbursement and lower the overall cost of healthcare. Hospital rate-setting was implemented under state law by the state cost review commission. The commissions in these states are responsible for establishing the maximum charge for each hospital service. Rate-setting was in effect for seven states for 14 years or more, but is in effect currently in only two states: Maryland (General Assembly of Maryland, n.d.) and West Virginia (West Virginia Code, Chapter 16, §16-29B-1 et seq., n.d.) (Atkinson, G., 2009).

CMS has previously denied provider-based status based on the determination of a state cost review commission. CMS denied provider-based status for an emergency department operated by Shady Grove Adventist Hospital nine miles away in Germantown, Maryland, based on a determination by a state cost review commission. In that case, the Maryland Health Services Cost Review Commission (HSCRC) ruled that it had no authority to regulate the services furnished at the Germantown Emergency Center, but it did not take any position as to whether the center was provider-based under federal regulations (In the Case of Shady Grove, 2008).

Shady Grove submitted an attestation to CMS for approval of provider-based status for the emergency center. CMS determined that the Germantown Emergency Center met all of the requirements at 42 *CFR* §413.65 (2011) for provider-based status as a remote location of the Shady Grove Hospital, except the criteria at 42 *CFR* §413.65(d)(1) (2011). CMS denied provider-based status for the emergency center based on its conclusion that the Maryland HSCRC did not consider the center to be part of Shady Grove, the main provider, for state rate-setting purposes. Specifically, Highmark, the MAC for Shady Grove, determined that "the Maryland HSCRC 'does not consider a facility which is not physically adjacent to a hospital to be part of the hospital' " (In the Case of Shady Grove, 2008). CMS concluded that "the Commission has found that the facility is not providing 'hospital services' and therefore it does not meet the 42 *CFR* §413.65(d)(1) requirement" (In the Case of Shady Grove, 2008).

CMS stated in its notice of denial that:

> *"It has long been the position of CMS that it would be inappropriate for a facility*
> *to be considered separate from the main provider, i.e., not provider-based, for state*
> *rate-setting purposes in those states that have a cost review commission or other*

agency that has the authority to regulate facility reimbursement while, at the same time, claiming provider-based status for Medicare purposes."

—In the Case of Shady Grove, 2008.

While the ALJ overturned CMS' determination, the ALJ's decision was reversed by the Appellate Division of the DAB, which upheld CMS' interpretation of the regulation (Shady Grove Adventist Hospital, 2008). The Appellate Division concluded that the HSCRC made the requisite finding that the emergency center was not part of the Shady Grove Hospital, which meant that it does not qualify as provider-based under 42 *CFR* §413.65(d)(1) (2011).

Clinical integration

Central to the concept of provider-based billing is the requirement that the provider-based departments be clinically integrated with the main hospital provider (42 *CFR* §413.65[d][2], 2011). This means that the hospital treats the clinical services furnished in the provider-based department exactly the same as the services furnished in all of the other hospital departments, regardless of location. From the perspective of the hospital, this helps to ensure that the hospital is able to guarantee the same quality of care in all of its hospital outpatient departments. From the patient's perspective, this means that patients should have the same care experience in all of the hospital departments. When examined from this perspective, it is much easier to understand why CMS is so invested in enforcing these requirements.

Hospitals should also be interested in maintaining the quality of their brand across any location that displays the hospital name, including the provider-based departments, both on- and off-campus. In effect, because of this clinical integration, the hospital is guaranteeing that a patient's experience is identical in any of the hospital departments, and the transition between the various hospital departments is seamless and easy to negotiate.

CMS expects to find clinical integration in the following six areas:

- **Professional staff.** One of the key controls hospitals have over clinical quality is the ability to require that physicians and other professionals obtain clinical privileges through the hospital medical staff prior to furnishing services to hospital patients. This function is also required under the Medicare hospital *CoPs* (42 *CFR* §482.12[a], 2011; 42 *CFR* §482.22, 2011). Therefore, it makes sense that CMS requires that the professionals who furnish services in a provider-based department have clinical privileges at the main hospital provider (42 *CFR* §413.65[d][2][i], 2011). In order to meet this requirement, the hospital should ensure that the medical staff office utilizes the same process to grant clinical privileges to new physicians requesting to practice in any hospital outpatient location, including the physicians practicing in provider-based departments. In addition, the medical staff should require the same periodic recredentialing process, and subject the provider-based physicians to the same medical staff bylaws, rules, and regulations as all of the other medical staff members.

If CMS or its contractor audits this requirement, it would expect to find the hospital-based physician credentialing files in the same location as all of the other medical staff files. In addition, the expectation is that the forms used to perform the credentialing and the documents collected during the process should be the same. Finally, the credentialing decisions should be reviewed by the same medical staff committee and through the same process as physicians in other departments.

As with other provider-based requirements, hospitals that build provider-based departments at the same time as the main hospital, or under the same long-term planning process, are less likely to have difficulties in meeting this requirement. In that case, the hospital is already likely to be partnering with the physicians in these locations, and the physicians are already well-integrated into the hospital medical staff process. However, when a freestanding physician office or other entity is acquired long after the hospital is built, the hospital medical staff is more likely to neglect the integration of these new physicians into the medical staff credentialing process. In addition, the physicians practicing in the provider-based department are less likely to easily accept the need to comply with the hospital credentialing process, given their history of practicing in a more independent fashion.

- **Monitoring and oversight.** Hospitals are required to monitor and oversee the quality of care furnished to patients through various mechanisms. Many of these requirements are imposed on hospitals by licensing and accrediting bodies. For example, hospitals are required by CMS and accrediting bodies to operate performance improvement, utilization management, incident reporting, and other similar processes (42 *CFR* §482.21, 2011). These requirements serve to monitor and improve the care furnished by physicians, nurses, technicians, and other healthcare practitioners at the hospital.

  In order to ensure that the quality of care furnished in provider-based departments is equivalent to the care provided at the main hospital, CMS requires that the provider-based departments be subjected to the same oversight and monitoring as all other hospital departments (42 *CFR* §413.65[d][2][ii], 2011). For example, the provider-based departments must conduct performance improvement monitoring and remediation targeted at the specific type of services furnished there. Again, it is in the best interest of hospitals to ensure that all of its departments, including on- and off-campus provider-based departments, are held to the same high expectations to ensure that the care delivered under the hospital's name is uniform throughout the facility.

- **Medical staff committees.** Once physicians are credentialed at a hospital, the hospital exercises oversight and control over the quality of medical care through its bylaws, rules, and regulations, as well as various medical staff committees, including quality assurance, utilization management, peer review, infection control, and mortality and morbidity review (42 *CFR* §482.12[a], 2011; 42 *CFR* §482.22, 2011). The medical staff also operates various department committees to set standards for and to review clinical practice. These include departmental committees for surgery, medicine, pediatrics, OB/GYN, and emergency medicine, among others.

  Similar to the monitoring and oversight expected of the hospital and medical staff credentialing discussed above, CMS demands that the medical staff in all hospital departments be subjected to the oversight of the medical staff committees (42 *CFR* §413.65[d] [2][iv], 2011). Again, this expectation seems to be in the best interest of the hospital, so patients can expect the same level of scrutiny of medical practice throughout the facility and not worry that care furnished in provider-based departments is inferior.

- **Medical director reporting relationship.** Hospitals are required by state and federal law, as well as accrediting bodies, to have a chief medical officer or similar officer to oversee the physician services furnished in the hospital (42 *CFR* §482.21[e], 2011). The various medical departments and facilities that furnish these services generally also have medical directors to manage the medical care in each of these departments. For example, the radiology, pathology, laboratory, OB/GYN, pediatrics, oncology, radiation therapy, surgery, and medical departments all have chiefs or medical directors who develop and monitor the standards of clinical care in these specialized medical fields.

  Similar to many of the other provider-based requirements, the hospital must ensure that the medical directors of all of the provider-based departments have the same reporting relationship to the chief medical officer as the other hospital departments. In addition, the medical directors of provider-based departments should be under the same type of supervision and accountability as any other director, medical or otherwise (42 *CFR* §413.65[d][2][iii], 2011). For example, if surgical procedures are performed in a provider-based department, those services should not only be subjected to the scrutiny of the medical staff committee structure, but should also be furnished under the same clinical guidelines and other standards established by the main hospital's chief of surgery. If the provider-based radiation oncology department has its own medical director, then he or she should report up to the hospital's chief hematology/oncology medical director. This reporting relationship should be expressly reflected in the medical staff organizational chart, rather than just exist in the minds of the physicians.

- **Unified retrieval system for medical records.** Whether the medical records are maintained in a paper or electronic format, the hospital must ensure the records generated to document services furnished in the provider-based departments are accessible through a unified retrieval system along with all of the other hospital records (42 *CFR* §413.65[d][2] [v], 2011). This is also required under the hospital *CoPs*:

"The hospital must use a system of author identification and record maintenance that ensures the integrity of the authentication and protects the security of all record entries."

—42 *CFR* 482.24(b), 2011.

This does not mean that the records are all maintained in exactly the same format in all of the hospital departments. CMS explained this requirement in the *Federal Register* discussion of these regulations:

"We would like to clarify that what is intended is that a system be maintained under which both the potential provider-based entity or department of a provider and the main provider have access to the beneficiary's record, so that practitioners in either location can obtain relevant medical information about care in the other setting."

—65 *Fed. Reg.* 18434, 18515, 2000.

For example, a provider-based clinic may have a simple paper medical record that is unique to that clinic, and the other hospital departments may have a more sophisticated electronic medical record (EMR). However, this will meet the provider-based requirements as long as the medical record number assigned to the patient in all of these locations is the same and the records are maintained in a centralized manner that makes them easily accessible throughout hospital facilities. In addition, these records must all be considered to comprise the unified medical record for a patient at the hospital.

The provider-based requirements would likely not be met if the provider-based department maintains its own separate medical record files for its patients. The same applies when: the patient has a medical record number in that department distinct from the medical record number assigned in other hospital departments, that department's medical record is not produced when the hospital medical record is requested, and/or there is no easy method of accessing that record. It would also be difficult (although not impossible) to ensure that the medical records are integrated if there is more than one person responsible for the various medical records and the records are stored separately, especially in off-campus departments located miles from the main hospital.

- **Outpatients have full access to care at main provider.** Similar to the requirement for a unified medical record, CMS requires integration of the inpatient and outpatient services at the hospital and the provider-based facility or unit (42 *CFR* §413.65[d][2][vi], 2011). This means that patients treated at the provider-based department who require further care have full access to the services furnished at the hospital. In addition, CMS would expect that the patients actually are referred to the main hospital for these inpatient and outpatient services.

CMS does not intend that patients be *forced* to obtain their care at the main hospital:

"[T]he commenter expressed concern about the potential impact of this section on a patient's freedom of choice. The commenter believes that the entity's efforts to meet this standard would limit a patient's freedom of choice. The commenter suggested that we clarify our position so that providers acting in good faith will not be sanctioned for attempting to comply with this requirement.

Response: Paragraph (d)(4)(vi) requires only that patients have access to the services of the main provider and that they be referred to it where the referral is appropriate. We wish to clarify that these criteria are not intended to restrict patient freedom of choice or the practitioner's freedom to refer patients to other locations, where doing so will result in better care for the patient."

—65 *Fed. Reg.* 18434, 18515–16, 2000.

This requirement, like many of the others, is easier to meet when the provider-based clinics were integrated when the hospital was built. This is true because the provider-based physicians tend to identify themselves more with the main hospital and are more likely to refer their clinic patients to the main hospital for inpatient services, rather than to other hospitals in which they may have medical staff privileges. Physicians in these hospitals are more likely to be invested in the hospital's mission and research and to identify closely with the hospital.

To the contrary, when a hospital acquires a freestanding clinic that was independently operated for many years, the physicians are more likely to have looser affiliations with the main hospital and are just as likely to refer patients to other hospitals as the main hospital. The hospital will have to educate the hospital-based physicians in those cases about the importance of referring patients to the hospital whenever possible and foster relationships with them to help them more closely identify with the hospital.

Financial integration

Just like the mandate for clinical integration, CMS expects the hospital to financially integrate the provider-based department with the remainder of the hospital's operation (42 *CFR* §413.65[d][3], 2011). This means that the hospital must report the provider-based department's income and expenses along with other hospital departments in any financial reports and audits. The hospital should assign a cost center to the provider-based department, and the general ledger for the provider-based department should roll up to that cost center on the income and expense reports for the hospital. Finally, the costs for the provider-based department should be reported on the hospital cost report under the cost center for the provider-based department. In effect, anyone reviewing the financial records for the hospital should see no appreciable difference between the reporting of income and expenses for the provider-based department and any other hospital department.

Public awareness

The previously discussed provider-based requirements are intended to ensure that the patient's experience once they arrive at the provider-based department is the same as they would have in any other hospital department. CMS also wants to ensure that there is no appreciable difference in how these departments appear to the public even before the patient opens the door to the clinic (42 *CFR* §413.65[d][4], 2011). This requirement is designed to guarantee that Medicare beneficiaries are given notice long before they request services that they are in a hospital outpatient department, rather than a freestanding physician office. Because of this notice, CMS hopes that the beneficiaries will not be surprised to receive bills from the hospital for facility services, rather than just expecting a professional bill from a freestanding physician office.

To accomplish this, the hospital should examine the building signage, website, answering machine message, business cards, and any other publicly-available documents for the provider-based department to ensure that the hospital name, logo, and other standard hospital messaging is present. Similarly, the hospital should educate the staff and physicians in the provider-based clinic to refer to the clinic as part of the hospital, rather than simply as the offices of the physicians who practice there.

As with many of these requirements, hospitals that have operated provider-based departments for many years will likely not have much trouble with this requirement. This is because these departments will likely be well integrated into the hospital's operations, and the public is more likely to readily identify these departments as part of the hospital. Hospitals that have more recently acquired provider-based departments are likely to find pockets of noncompliance with this requirement, because the clinic may still be using the website, business cards, signage, or other materials from its previous life as a freestanding clinic.

The importance of compliance with this requirement was recently examined by the DAB in Mercy Hospital Lebanon, *DAB Decision No. CR3320* (2014). In that case, CMS determined that a remote location of the Mercy Hospital Lebanon in Missouri did not meet provider-based requirements based on, among other things, the fact that the signage, website, and business cards found in the remote location did not have the same name as the main provider. This finding was overturned by the ALJ on appeal, based on a determination that the hospital was in the process of changing its name (Mercy Hospital Lebanon, 2014). However, this highlights the importance of this requirement and how closely CMS reviews it. Therefore, hospitals should closely audit requirements in these recently acquired departments, including opening cabinets and drawers to remove all old business cards, letterhead, educational materials, medical record forms, and signage to eliminate any possibility that the name and logo from the old clinic appears in front of the patients, rather than the hospital's name and logo.

Compliance with hospital Conditions of Participation, including Life Safety Code® provisions

It should go without saying that, as a hospital outpatient department, provider-based departments associated with hospitals must comply with all of the terms of the hospital's Medicare provider agreement, including all applicable Medicare hospital *CoPs* and other applicable laws (42 *CFR* §§413.65[d][5], [g][3], [g][8], 2011). This includes any National Fire Protection Association 101 *Life Safety Code*® provisions applicable to that type of hospital department. CMS mandates that all certified facilities comply with the *Life Safety Code* to ensure basic fire safety. (See discussion of CMS' use of the *Life Safety Code* provisions at *www.cms.gov/Medicare/Provider-Enrollment-and-Certification/CertificationandComplianc/LSC.html*.)

Basically, the provider-based department should just be one of the many hospital-based departments listed on the CMS 855A form that the hospital submits for CMS certification. In addition, it should be treated the same as any other hospital department during the survey and certification process. If the hospital applies for deemed status through the Joint Commission or another accrediting body, the provider-based department should be surveyed and accredited by the same organization, rather than being accredited through another organization. This does not preclude the hospital from obtaining specialized certification or accreditation for certain services in addition to the main Medicare certification.

When a hospital opens or acquires a new hospital-based department, the first step it should take after putting the department on the hospital license is to send a revised 855A to its MAC with all of the information necessary to add the new department under the hospital's Medicare provider number. This includes the name of the service as well as the actual address of the department, because this is often different from the main hospital address. Also, the hospital should ensure that this information is updated whenever the department relocates. This is the easiest requirement for CMS to audit and, hence, one of the first and easiest places to find errors.

After enrolling the provider-based department on the 855A, the harder task is ensuring that the department actually meets the hospital *CoPs* for the identified service type. Again, compliance with this requirement is more difficult when the hospital has recently acquired freestanding physician offices, because the office space is less likely to meet any applicable *Life Safety Code* provisions, and the staff is less likely to have been trained in compliance with the hospital *CoPs*.

© 2015 HCPro

A significant amount of education will be necessary for the staff, and there may be substantial construction or other effort necessary to meet the *CoPs* in these areas.

Correct billing for physician services

One of the biggest differences between provider-based departments and freestanding physician offices is the method of billing for the services. As discussed in more detail in Chapter 6, in a freestanding physician office, the professional services are billed on a CMS 1500 form (837P electronic form) with POS code 11, which indicates that the services were furnished in a physician office setting (*Medicare Claims Processing Manual*, Chapter 26. §10.5, 2014). When the professional services are billed with POS code 11, CMS does not expect to receive a separate bill from a hospital for provider-based facility services. Therefore, this triggers the MAC to pay the professional services based on the full MPFS amount for these services.

In contrast, in a provider-based clinic, there are generally two claims generated for the services:

- A claim from the physician for professional services on a CMS 1500 form (837P electronic form) with the POS code 22 (effective in 2016, POS 22 or 19), which signifies that the professional services were performed in a hospital outpatient department

- A claim from the hospital on a UB-04 Uniform Bill (837I electronic form) for the facility services performed in the hospital outpatient department

Again, as discussed in more detail in Chapter 6, the payment for the professional services is generally lower in this case, because the facility portion of the payment is reserved for the hospital facility claim. Submission of the POS code 22 (effective in 2016, POS 22 or POS 19) on the professional claim triggers this reimbursement methodology and allows the MAC to correctly calculate the payment for the professional services.

If a hospital is operating a provider-based clinic, it must work closely with the entity that is generating the claims for the professional services furnished in that clinic to ensure that the POS code on those claims is 22, rather than 11. If the professional claims are generated with POS code 11 instead of 22, the hospital may be found out of compliance with the provider-based requirements for that clinic (42 *CFR* §413.65[g][2], 2011).

Nondiscrimination provisions

CMS requires that physicians who work in hospital outpatient departments comply with the nondiscrimination requirements of 42 *CFR* §489.10(b) (2003) (42 *CFR* 413.65[g][4], 2011). In particular, in order to participate in the Medicare program, the hospital (and, hence, the physicians who practice there) must meet the applicable civil rights requirements of:

1. *"Title VI of the Civil Rights Act of 1964, as implemented by 45 CFR part 80, which provides that no person in the United States shall, on the ground of race, color, or national origin,*

> *be excluded from participation in, be denied the benefits of, or be subject to discrimination under, any program or activity receiving Federal financial assistance (section 601);*
>
> 2. *Section 504 of the Rehabilitation Act of 1973, as implemented by 45 CFR part 84, which provides that no qualified handicapped person shall, on the basis of handicap, be excluded from participation in, be denied the benefits of, or otherwise be subject to discrimination under any program or activity receiving Federal financial assistance;*
>
> 3. *The Age Discrimination Act of 1975, as implemented by 45 CFR part 90, which is designed to prohibit discrimination on the basis of age in programs or activities receiving Federal financial assistance. The Age Discrimination Act also permits federally assisted programs and activities, and beneficiaries of Federal funds, to continue to use certain age distinctions, and factors other than age, that meet the requirements of the Age Discrimination Act and 45 CFR part 90; and*
>
> 4. *Other pertinent requirements of the HHS Office of Civil Rights."*
>
> *—42 CFR §489.10(b), 2003.*

Just like with any other department, the hospital must ensure that the phsicians in the provider-based departments also comply with these same nondiscrimination provisions (42 *CFR* §413.65[g][4], 2011). In order to accomplish this, the hospital should implement the same orientation and annual education program regarding these requirements with the provider-based physicians as it does with all of its other hospital physicians and staff.

Treat all patients as hospital outpatients

Although this may seem obvious from the discussion about the other provider-based requirements, CMS separately prohibits hospital-based departments from billing some Medicare beneficiaries as physician office patients and others as hospital-based patients. This rule does not apply to RHCs. In addition, CMS does recognize that this same limitation does not necessarily apply to patients insured by commercial payers (42 *CFR* §413.65[g][5], 2011). In other words, a hospital could establish a method of billing some patients with commercial coverage in hospital-based departments as if the services were furnished in a freestanding physician office. In that case, the hospital must also take steps to segregate these services on the Medicare cost report.

The hospital should work closely with its MAC and the commercial payers in establishing any such disparate billing methodologies, because this can be very confusing to the billing staff and physicians. If this requirement is audited, the hospital would want to ensure that the hospital-based physicians and patient financial services staff do not accidentally bill the Medicare patients incorrectly or misstate these requirements.

 © 2015 HCPro

Three-day payment window

For purposes of payment of inpatient hospital services furnished to Medicare beneficiaries, certain outpatient services provided to the patient by the hospital within three days prior to an inpatient admission are considered to be covered costs of the inpatient admission. This billing and payment rule, which is applicable to CAHs as well as hospitals subject to IPPS, is commonly referred to as the three-day payment window. Hospitals that are not CAHs or not subject to IPPS are required to comply with a similar one-day payment window, which bundles payment for outpatient services furnished by the hospital one day before the admission with the payment for the inpatient services (*Medicare Claims Processing Manual*, Chapter 3, §40.3, 2014).

Some services are excluded from the three-day and one-day payment windows, including services not subject to OPPS, physician professional services, non-covered services, and certain therapeutic services furnished within the payment window. (See 42 *CFR* §412.2[c][5], 2011; *Medicare Claims Processing Manual*, Chapter 3, §40.3, 2014.) We will not cover these exclusions in detail here.

Under the three-day payment window, the hospital is required to combine the charges from the outpatient visit with the inpatient claim and may not submit a separate outpatient claim type for these services. As a result, the IPPS hospital receives only the inpatient diagnosis-related group (DRG) payment for the entire encounter, rather than an OPPS payment for the outpatient services and a separate DRG payment for the inpatient services. Under this billing and payment rule, CAHs receive one payment for all of the inpatient and outpatient services based on the inpatient reasonable cost methodology for CAHs, rather than separate inpatient and outpatient payments.

The only services that hospitals must bundle under the three-day and one-day payment windows are outpatient services furnished by the same hospital to which the patient was admitted as an inpatient, i.e., any entity that is "wholly owned or operated by the hospital," and preadmission services furnished "by another entity under arrangements with the hospital." This includes outpatient services furnished by any hospital department, including both on- and off-campus provider-based departments (42 *CFR* §412.2[c][5], 2011; *Medicare Claims Processing Manual*, Chapter 3, §40.3, 2014).

Based on the rules stated above, it is understandable that CMS also expects that a hospital must ensure it complies with the three-day payment window for all of the services furnished by its hospital-based clinics in order for these clinics to be approved as provider-based (42 *CFR* §413.65[g][6], 2011). If the hospital neglects this requirement and allows the outpatient services furnished in its hospital-based clinics to be billed separately when a patient is admitted to the main hospital within the applicable payment window, CMS is likely to find that the clinic is not really being operated as a provider-based entity. Therefore, the hospital should carefully review its billing processes to ensure that it is able to accurately identify when outpatient services subject to the payment window have been furnished in all of its provider-based clinics, both on- and off-campus. The hospital must then create manual or electronic billing processes to ensure that no outpatient claim is submitted for those services, and they are instead bundled into the inpatient hospital claim. This may be difficult in those hospital-based clinics that have previously utilized separate billing personnel to submit claims for those outpatient services. The hospital will have to closely review its billing systems and practices to integrate the billing in a compliant fashion.

EMTALA (anti-dumping) compliance

As a condition of participation in the Medicare program, hospitals with emergency departments must comply with the anti-dumping provisions of 42 *CFR* §§489.20(l), (m), (q), and (r) (2011), and 43 *CFR* §489.24(b), which were implemented as a result of the Emergency Medical Treatment and Active Labor Act (EMTALA), Section 1867 of the Social Security Act. As an integral part of the hospital, any on-campus hospital-based departments must also comply with this law just like all other on-campus hospital departments (42 *CFR* §413.65[g][1][i], 2011). However, this law does not apply to off-campus hospital-based departments, except for off-campus dedicated emergency departments as defined in 42 *CFR* §489.24(b) (2014) (42 *CFR* §413.65[g][1][ii], 2011).

In order to comply with EMTALA, if a person presents to the hospital's dedicated emergency department—on hospital property or in any hospital-based department—the hospital must provide an appropriate medical screening examination within the capability of its emergency department to determine whether an emergency medical condition exists. In addition, if an emergency medical condition is determined to exist, the hospital must provide any necessary stabilizing treatment or an appropriate transfer as defined in the law. This medical screening exam and stabilizing treatment must be accomplished prior to inquiring about the patient's insurance status or ability to pay. This law also requires the following:

- EMTALA signage/posting requirements
- A list of on-call physicians
- A central log and records of transfers to and from the facility
- Reporting of inappropriate transfers from other facilities

Additional and More Stringent Rules That Apply to Off-Campus Provider-Based Departments

While CMS expects compliance by all provider-based departments, there is heightened concern about off-campus departments. As noted previously, any provider-based department located more than 250 yards from the hospital campus is considered to be off-campus. Because of the distance from the main hospital campus, these units are more likely to be mistaken by Medicare beneficiaries as freestanding physician offices and are also less likely to be integrated with the hospital clinical operations, as required by CMS. This also means that Medicare patients may be surprised to be charged both professional and hospital copayments for these services, rather than just the patient liability for the professional services. Therefore, while the off-campus provider-based departments must meet all of the other criteria already discussed in this chapter, CMS also expects off-campus departments to comply with the additional, more stringent requirements discussed below.

Written patient notice

Because off-campus provider-based departments are more likely to be viewed by Medicare beneficiaries as stand-alone physician offices, CMS requires these departments to furnish written notice to the beneficiary before the delivery of services. The notice must explain the beneficiary's financial liability, or:

> "If the exact type and extent of care needed are not known, an explanation that the beneficiary will incur a coinsurance liability to the hospital that he or she would not incur if the facility were not provider-based, an estimate based on typical or average charges for visits to the facility, and a statement that the patient's actual liability will depend upon the actual services furnished by the hospital."

> —42 CFR §413.65(g)(7)(i), 2011.

The notice "must be one that the beneficiary can read and understand" (42 CFR §413.65[g][7][ii], 2011). The notice may be furnished to the patient's authorized legal representative if the patient is unable to read it because he or she is unconscious, under great duress, or otherwise unable to read or understand the notice, as long as the notice is furnished prior to the delivery of services (42 CFR §413.65[g][7][iii], 2011). This notice should be furnished only after the patient is stabilized in accordance with the EMTALA rules discussed above, if the provider-based department is subject to that law (i.e., is an off-campus dedicated emergency department) (42 CFR §413.65[g][7][v], 2011).

This notice provides essential education for Medicare beneficiaries, especially in those situations when a hospital is acquiring a previously freestanding physician clinic. Provision of the notice along with a verbal explanation of the change in billing in the provider-based setting may decrease the number of concerns raised by Medicare beneficiaries in these situations. Hospitals should consider not only posting the notice in provider-based clinics, but also furnishing written notices prior to the patient's encounter. In addition, it is helpful to post the notice on the hospital's website, since this is often the first place that potential patients access information about the facility. Posting the notice online is also helpful in supporting the public image of the location as a provider-based facility. A good example of a required hospital notice to patients posted by St. Luke's University Health Network is found at *www.slhn.org/Pay-Bills/Hospital-Based-Provider-Based-Outpatient-Billing.*

Under ownership and control of main provider

Under the requirements listed above, it is clear that provider-based departments must be monitored and overseen by the main provider. However, because off-campus departments are more likely to be operated outside of the hospital's control, CMS requires even stricter integration for these departments. Specifically, these departments must be clearly operated under the ownership and control of the main provider, evidenced by the following:

1. The business entity that operates the off-campus facility is 100% owned by the main provider;

2. The main provider and the off-campus department have the same governing body;

3. The main provider and the off-campus department are operated under the same organizational documents, including the organizational bylaws; and

4. The main provider has final responsibility for administrative decisions, final approvals for contracts with outside parties, final approval for personnel actions, final responsibility for personnel policies (such as fringe benefits or code of conduct), and final approval for medical staff appointments in the facility or organization.

    —*42 CFR* §413.65(e)(1), 2011.

Administration and supervision

CMS also has enunciated stricter requirements for the administration and supervision of off-campus departments to ensure that they have exactly the same relationship with the main provider as other departments (42 *CFR* §413.65[e][2], 2011). These departments must be directly supervised by the main provider, have a direct reporting relationship with managers at the main provider, and be accountable to the governing body of the main provider in the same manner as other hospital departments. Services such as billing, medical records, human resources, payroll, employee salary and benefits, and purchasing must be completely integrated with the main provider. The same employees must handle these functions for both the main provider and the off-campus department. Alternatively, the services may be furnished by another entity under contract, as long as:

*   The services are furnished by the main provider and the off-campus department under the same contract agreement, or

*   The services are handled under different contracts, but are both managed by the main provider (42 *CFR* §413.65[e][2][iii], 2011)

Location

Hospitals may believe that they are able to control the operations of off-campus departments many miles from the main campus, especially given the marvels of modern technology and communication techniques. However, CMS believes that there are limitations to this ability based on the distance from the main provider and other factors. Therefore, CMS has defined the allowable locations for off-campus provider-based departments (42 *CFR* §413.65[e][3], 2011). First, the off-campus department must be in the same state as the main provider or, when consistent with the laws of both states, in adjacent states (42 *CFR* §413.65[e][3][iv], 2011). In addition, CMS also requires off-campus departments to meet one of the following requirements:

- The facility is within 35 miles of the main provider's campus (42 *CFR* §413.65[e][i], 2011)

- The facility is owned and operated by a hospital or CAH that has a disproportionate share adjustment (DSH) greater than 11.75%, or is a DSH hospital under 42 *CFR* §412.106(c)(2) (2011) operated by certain governmental agencies (42 *CFR* §413.65[e][3][ii], 2011)

- The facility serves the same patient population as the main provider, based on the past 12 months of patient encounters, in that:

  - At least 75% of the patients seen by the facility reside in same ZIP code as at least 75% of the patients served by the main provider, or

  - At least 75% of the patients seen in the provider-based department who need inpatient services obtain the services at the main provider (42 *CFR* §413.65[e][3][iii], 2011)

- The facility is an RHC that meets certain requirements (42 *CFR* §413.65(e)(3)(vi), 2011)

- The facility is a provider-based department located within specified distances from certain specialized providers (42 *CFR* §413.65(e)(3)(v), 2011)

The requirements regarding the location of off-campus provider-based departments are complex and must be reviewed in detail, especially if the entity is located further than 35 miles from the hospital campus. This requirement is explored in some detail in Mercy Hospital Lebanon, *DAB Decision No. CR3320* (2014). In that case, Mercy Hospital Lebanon operated a remote location of the hospital 55 miles away from the main hospital campus. Therefore, the location obviously failed to meet the less than 35 mile location criterion found at 42 *CFR* §413.65(e)(i) (2011). The ALJ also determined that the remote location failed to meet the criterion at 42 *CFR* §413.65(e)(ii) (2011). The main discussion in the case centered on whether the location met the criterion found at 42 *CFR* §413.65(e)(3)(iii) (2011), which would require that the remote location have a high level of integration with the main facility. The ALJ reviewed this criterion in detail and concluded that the facility served the same patient population as the main provider, based on the past 12 months of patient encounters, in that:

- At least 75% of the patients seen by the facility reside in same ZIP code as at least 75% of the patients served by the main provider, or

- At least 75% of the patients seen in the provider-based department who need inpatient services obtain the services at the main provider.

    —Mercy Hospital Lebanon, 2014.

Off-campus locations under management contracts

If the off-campus location is operated under a management contract or a management service agreement, CMS is even more concerned that the main provider is actually operating the facility as an integral part of its services. Hence, in addition to all of the other integration requirements already outlined above, CMS requires that:

1. The main provider employ the patient care staff at the provider-based location; and

2. The management contract is held by the main provider itself, not by a parent entity that has control over both the main provider and the provider-based entity.

    —42 *CFR* §413.65(h), 2011.

Joint ventures

Provider-based departments operated under joint ventures have other requirements (42 *CFR* §413.65[f], 2011). For an entity operated as a joint venture to be considered provider-based, it must:

1. Be partially owned by at least one of the providers in the joint venture;

2. Be located on the main campus of the same provider who is the partial owner;

3. Be provider-based to that one provider whose campus on which the entity is located.

These types of provider-based entities must also meet all of the other provider-based criteria discussed above (42 *CFR* §413.65[f], 2011). Because of the complexity of these arrangements, it is recommended that these arrangements be subjected to legal review.

Grandfathering of Provider-Based Facilities

When CMS first promulgated the provider-based regulations, it designed provisions to give some protection to entities treated by hospitals as provider-based at that time the regulations became effective:

"If a facility was treated as provider-based in relation to a hospital or CAH [critical access hospital] on October 1, 2000, it will continue to be considered provider-based in relation to that hospital or CAH until the start of the hospital's first cost reporting period beginning on or after July 1, 2003 ... For purposes of this paragraph (b)(2), a facility is considered as provider-based on October 1, 2000 if, on that date, it either had a written determination from CMS that it was provider-based, or was billing and being paid as a provider-based department or entity of the hospital."

—42 *CFR* 413.65(b)(2), 2011.

This section of the *Code of Federal Regulations (CFR)* is commonly referred to as a "grandfathering clause." All hospitals are past the point of being able to utilize this grandfathering provision because this grandfathering period has passed. Therefore, it has little effect on current provider-based status for hospital departments. However, as discussed in a later chapter, the grandfathering provision may assist in limiting the retroactive damages for any later determination of noncompliance under 42 *CFR* 413.65(j) (2011).

Scenarios

The following scenarios will assist in further understanding the criteria for provider-based status. In each of these scenarios, the following facts are assumed: ABC Hospital is owned by The Big Hospital Group along with several other hospitals in the area, and the compliance officer for ABC Hospital is auditing the hospital outpatient departments for compliance with the provider-based requirements.

Scenario A

One of the auditors finds the following:

The hospital neurology clinic is located in an adjacent medical office building on the hospital campus and is staffed with hospital employees. The clinic was previously freestanding and was purchased by the hospital last year. This clinic is directed by an administrative manager and a medical director. The neurologists in the clinic are not listed as having hospital medical staff privileges. The clinic is not listed on the organizational chart, and the manager reports only to the clinic medical director. The clinic medical director makes all of the decisions about standards of medical care and does not consult with the chief medical officer at ABC Hospital. The patients are registered and billed as hospital outpatients.

The auditor asks whether the clinic meets the provider-based criteria and, if not, which criteria are not met.

Response:

This clinic fails to meet the requirement under 42 *CFR* §413.65(d)(2)(i) (2011) that the professionals who furnish services in the provider-based department have medical staff privileges at the main hospital. In addition, the clinical services do not appear to be integrated with the main hospital in any other manner, as required by the regulations. The clinic manager does not report to the hospital, and the clinical services do not appear to be overseen by the hospital quality committees, as required by 42 *CFR* §413.65(d)(2)(ii) (2011). Finally, the medical director of the clinic does not report to the hospital CMO and the services are apparently not overseen by the hospital medical staff committe, as required by 42 *CFR* §§413.65(d)(2)(iii)–(iv) (2011).

The hospital should consult with legal counsel regarding potential self-disclosure and repayment due to this noncompliance (see Chapter 4).

Scenario B

When you call the neurology clinic discussed above to interview the clinic director, the clerk answers the phone, "Dr. Smith and Jones' office. May I assist you?" Curious, you pull up the hospital website and do not see the neurology clinic listed among the other hospital departments. In addition, when you do a search of the Internet, you find a clinic listed at that address called "Smith and Jones Neurology Clinic" with no reference to the hospital name.

Does this cause any additional problems meeting the provider-based clinic? If so, which criteria are not met?

Response:

This clinic fails to meet the public awareness criterion under 42 *CFR* §413.65(d)(4) (2011), because the clinic is not identified to the public in any manner as being part of ABC Hospital. To correct this, the staff must be educated to refer to the clinic as "ABC Hospital Neurology Clinic," the hospital website must be corrected to include the neurology clinic, and any old websites or references to the "Smith and Jones Neurology Clinic" must be deactivated.

The hospital should also consult with legal counsel regarding potential self-disclosure and repayment due to this noncompliance (see Chapter 4).

Scenario C

The auditor gives you a list of off-campus provider-based departments so that you can begin to visit each of them. You find the following in your on-site visits of some of these departments:

- The orthopedic clinic is located 30 miles from the hospital. You watch some of the patients being registered at the clinic. The registration clerk verbally states to each patient: "This clinic is part of ABC Hospital." No other notices are given to the patients or posted.

Response:

This clinic fails to meet the requirement under 42 *CFR* §413.65(g)(7) (2011) that *off-campus* provider-based departments provide written notice to Medicare beneficiaries that explains the beneficiary's financial liability to the hospital, because the services are furnished in a provider-based facility rather than a freestanding physician office. The verbal notice given is not sufficient to meet this requirement. To correct this, the hospital should either print written notices to be given to Medicare beneficiaries or post the notice in a location that is easily viewable by clinic patients. In addition, the hospital should educate the staff to be able to answer questions that may arise about this information.

The hospital should also consult with legal counsel regarding potential self-disclosure and repayment due to this noncompliance (see Chapter 4).

- The pediatrics clinic is located 10 miles from the main hospital and is operated under a management contract. You obtain the management contract and note that it was signed by the chief executive officer of Physician Management Company and the president of The Big Hospital Group. The management contract specifies that all of the managers, nurses, and medical assistants are leased employees (i.e., they are employees of Physician Management Company and not ABC Hospital). When you speak with the nurses in the clinic, they state that the location is a physician office and are surprised to learn that ABC Hospital owns the clinic.

Response:

This clinic fails to meet the requirements in 42 *CFR* §413.65(h) (2011) regarding off-campus provider-based departments operated under management contracts because:

   a) the management contract is signed by the parent organization of ABC Hospital, rather than ABC Hospital, as required; and

   b) the clinical staff in the clinic are employees of the management company, rather than ABC Hospital, as required.

To correct this, the management agreement must be renegotiated to have the clinical staff be employees of the hospital (the managers may remain as leased employees), and the new contract must be signed by ABC Hospital rather than the parent organization.

In addition, the clinical staff are violating the public awareness criterion under 42 *CFR* §413.65(d)(4) (2011) because the clinic is not identified to the public in any manner as being part of ABC Hospital. In fact, the clinical staff is totally unaware that the hospital operates the clinic. To correct this, the staff must be educated to refer to the clinic as "ABC Hospital Pediatrics Clinic."

The hospital should also consult with legal counsel regarding potential self-disclosure and repayment due to this noncompliance (see Chapter 4).

- The outpatient surgery department is down the street from the hospital. It was recently acquired from another company that was operating the location. The clinic has its own governing body and bylaws, and the policies and standardized procedures are different from the policies and procedures used at all of the other surgical clinics at ABC Hospital. The staff used to work for the other company and now are hospital employees. When you ask them questions about the clinic operations, they state that the clinic staff have more sick days granted to them than the staff at ABC Hospital, because these are the benefits that they had under the previous owner. They state that this decision was made by the outpatient surgery administrative director. Payroll for the surgical clinic is handled by a payroll company chosen by the outpatient surgery administrative director, and the contract for these services was also signed by that same director.

Response:

This clinic fails to meet the requirements found in 42 *CFR* §413.65(e)(1) (2011) that the off-campus department must have the same governing body and bylaws as the main hospital and that the main provider has the final authority to approve the employee benefits and contracts with outside entities. The use of the outside payroll company also violates the requirements in 42 *CFR* §413.65(e)(2) (2011) that the department must be supervised by the main provider and that services such as payroll are completely integrated with the main hospital. If payroll services are furnished under contract, they must be managed by the main provider, rather than the individual department. A complete reorganization and change in payroll companies is required to correct this situation.

In addition, the clinical services do not appear to be integrated with the main hospital, as required by the regulations. The clinic is operating under different clinical standards than the rest of the surgical clinics, and the clinical services do not appear to be overseen by the hospital quality committees, as required by 42 *CFR* §413.65(d)(2)(ii) (2011). The clinical standards must be revised and the staff must be educated in the revisions in order to correct this situation.

The hospital should also consult with legal counsel regarding potential self-disclosure and repayment due to this noncompliance (see Chapter 4).

- The Breast Center is located in a local shopping area a few miles from the hospital in space leased by the hospital. You review the billing that is done for the patients there and find that:

  a) The claims for professional services contain the POS code 11 for some Medicare patients and 22 (effective in 2016, POS 22 or 19) for others; and

  b) There are no hospital claims submitted for these services on a UB-04 claim form.

When you call the ABC Hospital controller, she is unable to give you the number of the cost center for the Breast Center and states that she was not told to include this location on the hospital cost report. She thinks that the clinic manages its own expenses and assets on a separate accounting record.

© 2015 HCPro

Response:

This clinic fails to meet the financial integration criterion found in 42 *CFR* §413.65(d)(3) (2011) that is required for all provider-based departments (not just for off-campus locations), because the clinic is not included on the ABC Hospital financial accounts or cost report. To correct this situation, the hospital must assign a cost center to this clinic, roll up the expenses and income from this department onto the hospital general ledger, and include the department in the hospital cost report.

The clinic is also violating the requirement for correct physician billing in 42 *CFR* §413.65(g)(2) (2011), which mandates that all physician billing for services furnished in the provider-based department contain the POS code 22 (effective in 2016, POS 22 or 19). In addition, the hospital is failing to comply with the requirement under 42 *CFR* §413.65(g)(5) that all of the Medicare patients be billed as hospital outpatients. To correct this situation, the hospital must work closely with the entity billing the physician services to ensure correct POS coding, and the hospital must begin registering and billing the Medicare patients as hospital outpatients.

The hospital should also consult with legal counsel regarding potential self-disclosure and repayment due to this noncompliance (see Chapter 4).

• You bring a copy of the hospital license with you and do not find any listing for the Diabetes Clinic that is three miles from the hospital campus. This clinic was acquired by the hospital three years ago. You call the hospital regulatory director, and she states that there was a letter sent to the state licensing agency when the clinic was acquired, requesting that the clinic be added to the hospital license. No response has been received, and no new license was issued. She states that she believes the clinic was added to the license, and, in any case, it does not matter because it definitely was added to the Medicare certification when she submitted a revised 855A form including this clinic.

Response:

This clinic fails to meet the requirement in 42 *CFR* §413.65(d)(1) for all provider-based departments that the clinic be included on the hospital license. It is appropriate that the clinic was added to the Medicare certification. However, that does not assist in complying with the licensure requirement. In addition, it does not meet the requirement simply to request that the clinic be added—the hospital must have in its hands the corrected license or other confirmation that the clinic was added to the license in order to comply with this requirement. To correct this, the hospital must immediately contact the licensing agency and ask for written confirmation that the clinic was added and the date of that addition.

The hospital should also consult with legal counsel regarding potential self-disclosure and repayment due to this noncompliance (see Chapter 4).

Provider-Based Determinations and Penalties for Failure to Meet Provider-Based Requirements

Enforcement of Provider-Based Requirements

There may be some hospital leaders who fail to take the provider-based requirements seriously. Some may even believe that CMS will not enforce these requirements, especially in those cases where the hospital has been operating a provider-based department for many years without any questions raised by the regulators. However, this could be a huge and costly mistake. To give you an idea how expensive this mistake could be, in a recent settlement agreement, Our Lady of Lourdes Memorial Hospital in Binghamton, New York, agreed to pay $3.3 million to settle its self-disclosed failure to comply with the provider-based requirements for a mobile hyperbaric center (Settlement Agreement Between United States of America and Our Lady of Lourdes Memorial Hospital, 2014). Our Lady of Lourdes billed for a hyperbaric center as though it was provider-based, even though it did not meet the criteria. In addition, the hospital had to self-disallow all of the costs for the hyperbaric center on all past cost reports for Medicare, Medicaid, TRICARE®, and Federal Employees Health Benefit Plan.

Not more than six months later, *AIS Health* reported in its Medicare Compliance Report that another hospital settled a similar case, again based on the failure to comply with the provider-based requirements for its hyperbaric center. In that case, W.A. Foote Memorial Hospital, doing business as Allegiance Health in Michigan, reportedly entered into a settlement agreement with the OIG and agreed to a $2.6 million civil monetary penalty for "improper payments from Medicare, Medicaid, and TRICARE for hyperbaric oxygen therapy services provided under a management agreement from October 10, 2008 to October 29, 2014" (Provider-Based Rules Trigger, 2014). Allegiance reportedly "self-disclosed these payments as a 'reportable event' under a corporate integrity agreement (CIA) that was already in place as part of the hospital's 2013 false claims settlement for improperly billed cardiovascular procedures and tests" ("Provider-Based Rules Trigger," 2014). (At the time of this writing, the settlement agreement for this case was not available.)

Providers cannot claim that they have not been previously warned to pay attention to the provider-based requirements. The OIG and CMS have sent numerous signals over the years that the government will aggressively seek out hospitals that are not in compliance with provider-based status. The 2005 OIG Supplemental Compliance Program Guidance for Hospitals noted that compliance with the provider-based requirements should be an integral part of hospitals' compliance plans:

> "*Improper claims for incorrectly designated 'provider-based' entities*
> *Certain hospital-affiliated entities and clinics can be designated as 'provider-based',*
> *which allows for a higher level of reimbursement for certain services. Hospitals*
> *should take steps to ensure that facilities or organizations are only designated as*
> *provider-based if they satisfy the criteria set forth in the regulations."*

> —*70 Fed. Reg. 4858, 2005.*

The OIG again warned hospitals in its 2014 and 2015 work plans that there are imminent plans to audit compliance with these requirements, given that there are higher payments for these services as compared to services furnished by freestanding clinics.

> "*Impact of provider-based status on Medicare billing policies and practices*
> *We will determine the impact of subordinate facilities in hospitals billing Medicare*
> *as being hospital-based (provider-based) and the extent to which such facilities meet*
> *CMS's criteria. Context—Provider-based status allows a subordinate facility to bill as*
> *part of the main provider. Provider-based status can result in additional Medicare*
> *payments for services furnished at provider-based facilities and may increase benefi-*
> *ciaries' coinsurance liabilities. In 2011, the Medicare Payment Advisory Commission*
> *(MedPAC) expressed concerns about the financial incentives presented by provid-*
> *er-based status and stated that Medicare should seek to pay similar amounts for*
> *similar services. (OEI; 04-12-00380; 04-12-00381; expected issue date: FY 2014; work*
> *in progress.)*

> *Comparison of provider-based and freestanding clinics (new) policies and practices*
> *We will review and compare Medicare payments for physician office visits in pro-*
> *vider-based clinics and freestanding clinics to determine the difference in payments*
> *made to the clinics for similar procedures and assess the potential impact on the*
> *Medicare program of hospitals' claiming provider-based status for such facilities.*

Context—Provider-based facilities often receive higher payments for some services than do freestanding clinics. The requirements to be met for a facility to be treated as a provider-based facility are at 42 CFR § 413.65(d). (OAS; W-00-14-35724; expected issue date: FY 2014; new start)."

—Office of Inspector General, 2014.

"Medicare oversight of provider-based status
We will determine the extent to which provider-based facilities meet CMS's criteria. Provider-based status allows facilities owned and operated by hospitals to bill as hospital outpatient departments. Provider-based status can result in higher Medicare payments for services furnished at provider-based facilities and may increase beneficiaries' coinsurance liabilities. In 2011, the Medicare Payment Advisory Commission (MedPAC) expressed concerns about the financial incentives presented by provider-based status and stated that Medicare should seek to pay similar amounts for similar services. (OEI; 04-12-00380; expected issue date: FY 2015)

Comparison of provider-based and freestanding clinics
We will review and compare Medicare payments for physician office visits in provider-based clinics and freestanding clinics to determine the difference in payments made to the clinics for similar procedures and assess the potential impact on the Medicare program of hospitals' claiming provider-based status for such facilities. Provider-based facilities often receive higher payments for some services than do freestanding clinics. The requirements to be met for a facility to be treated as provider-based are at 42 CFR § 413.65(d). (OAS; W-00-14-35724; W-00-15-35724; expected issue date: FY 2015)."

—Office of Inspector General, 2015.

How Does CMS Become Aware That a Hospital Is Operating Provider-Based Departments?

Hospital leaders may naively believe that CMS has no definite method of ascertaining that the hospital is operating a specific provider-based department. However, there are several ways in which CMS may become aware that a hospital is operating a provider-based department.

First, hospitals are required to submit annual cost reports that list the cost centers and departments operated by the hospital. CMS may become aware of a provider-based department's existence by examining these cost reports, especially in instances where the department is housed in buildings outside of the main hospital, because the addresses of these departments may be disclosed on the cost report. Based on that disclosure, CMS may begin an audit of the use of that provider-based department for that cost-reporting period and all prior periods.

CMS may also become aware of provider-based departments through routine certification and recertification surveys, even those performed through deemed status accreditation agencies like the Joint Commission. When completing those surveys, the hospital is required to list the departments/units that are to be included in the survey process, which would (and should) include a list of provider-based departments and their addresses. CMS may also conduct complaint surveys submitted by patients who received services furnished in the provider-based departments, and thus become aware that the hospital is furnishing services in a certain location. Based on that, CMS may conduct audits of the use of that provider-based department in all prior periods.

CMS also receives notification that the hospital is operating a provider-based department if the hospital decides to submit a voluntary attestation for that department. Hospitals expect that CMS will scrutinize the operations of the provider-based department beginning on the date of the attestation. They may not be aware, however, that CMS will not limit its scrutiny to the department's operations after the date of the voluntary attestation. Instead, CMS very well may audit the use of the department for cost-reporting periods prior to the date of the attestation.

As discussed more in depth in Chapter 5, beginning on January 1, 2016, CMS requires that main providers add a -PO informational modifier on each line of the UB-04 Uniform Bill claim form for services furnished in off-campus provider-based departments. CMS may learn of the existence of off-campus provider-based departments for the first time when the hospital begins to bill for services furnished in those departments using this -PO modifier. This, in fact, is one of the main purposes of this new requirement—to give CMS a readily available list of off-campus provider-based departments in order to audit compliance in those departments.

What Happens When CMS Becomes Aware of the Hospital's Provider-Based Departments?

A hospital may operate a specific provider-based department for many years, even decades, without undergoing a CMS audit of that department, which may lead to a false sense of security for the hospital leadership. However, CMS has the authority to audit that department at any time, even if a provider-based department was originally grandfathered into the program (42 *CFR* §413.65[b][2], 2011). As discussed, a CMS audit of the department's operations may lead to harsh financial penalties for the hospital if the provider-based requirements are not met.

 © 2015 HCPro

Audit based on submission of a voluntary attestation

CMS may also institute an audit when a hospital submits an attestation with its request to designate a location as a provider-based department. This requirement has changed over time, but submission of an attestation is now voluntary. Although it is voluntary and may lead to more scrutiny of the operation of the department, there are benefits to the submission of this attestation. The following concepts are important with relation to voluntary attestations:

- **History of voluntary attestations.** For years, hospitals operated provider-based departments with no specific CMS oversight or guidance. However, in a final rule published in April 2000, CMS implemented standard requirements for approval of provider-based requirements (65 *Fed. Reg.* 18504, 2000). Under those rules, attestations were *mandated* for a hospital to operate *all* provider-based departments that were not grandfathered under the regulations.

  However, as might be expected, CMS soon became overwhelmed with attestations for provider-based departments and requests for CMS determinations soon outstripped CMS' ability to issue these determinations in a timely fashion. As a consequence, in the latest provider-based regulation promulgated August 1, 2002, CMS lessened the restrictions and made the attestations for provider-based departments completely voluntary (42 *CFR* §413.65[b][3][i], 2011).

  CMS published *Transmittal A-03-030* in 2003 to implement the requirements under 42 *CFR* §413.65. According to that transmittal:

  "Effective October 1, 2002, the mandatory requirement for provider-based determinations under 42 CFR §413.65(b) (2011) was replaced with a voluntary attestation process. Providers are no longer required to apply for and receive a provider-based determination for their facilities prior to billing for services in those facilities as provider-based. However, under 42 CFR §413.65(b)(3) (2011), a provider may choose to obtain a determination of provider-based status by submitting an attestation stating that the facility meets the relevant provider-based requirements (depending on whether the facility is located on campus or off campus). Providers who wish to obtain such a determination of provider-based status for their facilities after October 1, 2002, should do so through the self-attestation process."

  —Transmittal A-03-030, Section B.1, 2003.

  "As noted above, facilities treated as provider-based in relation to a provider on October 1, 2000, are not affected by the revised regulations until the main provider's first cost reporting period starting on or after July 1, 2003. In the case of these

grandfathered facilities, any attestation regarding provider-based status will be considered only with respect to periods on or after that effective date."

—*Transmittal A-03-030*, Section B.1, 2003 (see also 42 *CFR* 413.65[b][2], 2011).

- **Details about voluntary attestations.** CMS has not published any official provider-based attestation form. However, it published a sample format outline for the attestation in *Transmittal A-03-030* (2003) (see Figure 4.1 at the end of this chapter). CMS states that providers "may use a letter, memo, or any other format that contains the necessary information instead of the Sample Form" (*Transmittal A-03-030*, Section B.5, 2003). According to the transmittal:

"At a minimum, the attestation should include:

- *The identity of the main provider and the facilities or organizations for which provider-based status is being sought*

- *An enumeration of each facility and a statement of its exact location (that is, its street address and whether it is on campus or off campus)*

- *Supporting documentation for off-campus facilities for purposes of applying the provider-based status criteria in effect at the time the request or attestation is submitted*

- *Information on the person to contact should CMS or the intermediary have further questions"*

—*Transmittal A-03-030*, Section B.6, 2003.

If the MAC for the hospital has published an attestation form, the hospital should use that form. Noridien offers the CMS sample form on its website (*www.noridianmedicare.com/provider/updates/docs/parta_attestation_form.pdf*). Cahaba Government Benefit Administrations, LLC, Palmetto GBA, and Wisconsin Physicians Services furnish slightly modified versions of this same attestation on their websites, some with more information than others (*www.cahabagba.com/documents/2012/02/part-a-enroll_attest.pdf, www.palmettogba.com/Palmetto/Providers.nsf/files/Provider_Based_Attestation_Statement_Revised_08062010.pdf/$FIle/Provider_Based_Attestation_Statement_Revised_08062010.pdf*, and *www.wps-medicare.com/j8macparta/departments/audit_reimbursement/_files/wps_attest_form.pdf*).

Documentation is required to be maintained for all items on the attestation, and certain information must actually be submitted with the attestation (42 *CFR* §413.65[b][3], 2011; *Transmittal A-03-030*, Section B.6, 2003). The main provider must submit documentation to support each requirement for an off-campus provider-based department. The hospital is not required to submit any documentation to support the attestation for on-campus provider-based departments, although submission of the supporting documentation is highly recommended. In particular, it may be helpful to submit a map of the campus. Even if the hospital decides not to submit the documentation, support for the attestation must be kept on file and furnished to CMS and the MAC upon request.

Before submitting an attestation, the hospital leadership should be reminded that an attestation is a legal document that can be used against it in a potential lawsuit. If the statements made on the attestation incorrectly describe the relationship between the hospital and the provider-based department, and payments are made to the hospital based on these statements, there may be liability under various state and federal laws, including the Health Insurance Portability and Accountability Act (HIPAA), Pub. Law No. 104–191, §§242-245, et seq., and the Federal False Statements Statute, 18 U.S.C. §1001. The Federal False Claims Statute prohibits, among other things, making false statements or concealing material facts in connection with the delivery of or payment for healthcare benefits. Therefore, it goes without saying that leadership should carefully review the statements made on the attestation and compare them against the actual operations of the provider-based department to ensure that all statements made are accurate and complete (omissions could be just as actionable as inaccurate statements in this context).

The attestation and all attached documentation should be submitted to the MAC, and an identical copy should be sent to the CMS RO (*Transmittal A-03-030* Section B.4, 2003). The MAC and/or RO is required to send the hospital written acknowledgment of receipt of the attestation after submission by the hospital (42 *CFR* §§413.65[b][3][iii] and [iv], 2011; *Transmittal A-03-030*, Section E.5, 2003). CMS then reviews the submission for completeness and consistency with the provider-based criteria, the documentation submitted with the attestation and with the information in the possession of CMS at the time the attestation is received. CMS then makes a determination as to whether the department is provider-based (42 *CFR* §413.65[a][3][iv], 2011). Note that in this regard, in making a determination, CMS presumes that an off-campus department that furnishes services of the kind ordinarily furnished in physician offices is a freestanding facility, unless proven otherwise by the hospital (42 *CFR* §413.65[b][4], 2011).

While the MAC may make the provider-based determination, the RO should approve or disapprove the application. Note that there is no mandatory deadline for CMS to respond to a hospital's provider-based submission. Therefore, depending on the MAC and RO, the issuance of a determination may take a significant period of time. The hospital should stay on top of the process and make periodic inquiries to ensure that the MAC/RO has not lost the submission and to minimize any potential delays. In addition, the hospital should ensure that it does not assume that the department will be approved—the hospital may consider not billing Medicare for newly acquired departments as provider-based until the determination has been received, especially for off-campus departments.

If the provider is denied provider-based status based on the attestation, the provider should respond to the determination as outlined below. In addition, the provider may request that CMS reconsider a determination that it does not qualify for provider-based status, and may appeal an adverse reconsideration decision before an ALJ of the DAB under the provisions of 42 *CFR* Part 498 (2011).

Hospitals that have submitted provider-based attestations may also report to CMS any material changes in the operations of the department, including a change of ownership or entry into a new or different management contract that would affect the provider-based determination (42 *CFR* §413.65[c], 2011). CMS may then take that opportunity to review the revised information for continued compliance with the provider-based requirements.

- **To submit or not to submit.** There are several benefits to submitting a voluntary attestation and obtaining a CMS determination for a provider-based department. First, preparing to obtain such a determination forces the hospital to closely examine its operations and ensure that it meets the provider-based requirements for each of its outpatient departments. Even if the hospital believed it operated its departments in accordance with the CMS requirements prior to preparing to submit the attestation, leadership will likely be surprised by what they discover when reviewing the details of their operations. Submission of the attestation puts the hospital operations into sharper focus and may lead to remediation of noncompliant practices simply by putting that department under the compliance microscope. During that process, the hospital may decide not to submit an attestation for specific departments after determining that the department should instead be treated as freestanding.

Receipt of a CMS provider-based determination also serves to decrease the uncertainty about how CMS will rule on compliance for the hospital departments, especially for off-campus provider-based departments. If CMS questions the documentation submitted, then the hospital may supplement the documentation, remediate its operations, or make a decision not to operate that department as provider-based. If CMS grants a provider-based determination, this decreases the risk that CMS will later rule that this is a freestanding entity, especially for off-campus departments for which full documentation is submitted. If the hospital continues to operate these departments in the same manner after receipt of the determination, the risk of a finding of noncompliance in the future is very remote.

There is another financial benefit to submission of an attestation. Even if CMS denies the attestation, the mere submission of the attestation serves to limit the recoupment of provider-based payments (*Transmittal A-03-030*, Section B.3, 2003). In that case, the recoupment starts only after the date the attestation was submitted, even if that is the same attestation that was denied, causing the recoupment to be incurred.

Of course, a hospital that submits a voluntary attestation should expect—and is in fact inviting—a detailed review of the provider-based department upon submission of that attestation. The hospital must submit documentation to support the requirements attested to for any off-campus provider-based department. In that case, CMS will review the documentation submitted and can be expected to challenge any documentation that does not support the provider-based requirements. In addition, CMS may request or seek out further information to support any requirements that are not already supported in the documentation submitted by the hospital or to further verify the hospital's operations. For example, if the hospital attests that the provider-based department is held out to the public as part of the hospital, CMS may independently review easily accessible materials such as the department's website, signage, publicly filed documents, and business cards to look for any information that contradicts the hospital's attestation.

Even if the hospital believes that it has remediated the department's operations in preparation for the submission of the attestation, the hospital should also anticipate and prepare itself for the fact that the submission of the attestation could lead to an audit of cost-reporting years prior to the date of the attestation. In that case, CMS has the authority to make an adverse determination based on the prior operation and billing for services in the provider-based department and recoup payments for those services as discussed in more detail below. This is more likely where the hospital has billed for a large volume of services or for costly services in that department for a number of years prior to submission of the attestation.

Initiation of an audit not based on voluntary attestation

If the hospital chooses not to submit a voluntary attestation and CMS receives notice of the provider-based department through the other methods detailed above (e.g., cost reports, surveys, and submission of the –PO modifier), CMS may begin an audit of that department at any time. Of course, CMS may also audit the operations of any provider-based department at any time, even if the provider has previously submitted an attestation. The first step that CMS will likely take in that case is to determine whether the hospital submitted an attestation for that department in the past. If that occurred, CMS will likely begin with the documentation submitted with that attestation—especially if dealing with an off-campus department—and will start its investigation with a comparison of the current operations with the hospital's previously submitted statements.

What are the penalties for failure to meet the provider-based rules?

If CMS determines that a hospital-based department fails to meet the provider-based requirements, CMS is required to first issue a notice to the hospital, indicating which cost-reporting periods are at risk in its determination. In the notice, CMS will indicate that it will:

1. *"Immediately adjust any future payments for the department/entity at issue to be paid at a freestanding entity rate;*

2. *Offer the hospital the opportunity to seek provider-based status for the department or continue to operate the unit as a separate freestanding unit; and*

3. *Recoup all payments paid at the higher provider-based rate for the cost reporting years identified in the Notice."*

   —42 CFR §413.65(j)(5), 2011

Under 42 *CFR* §413.65(j) (2011), the hospital has two potential pathways to take at this point:

- **Hospital responds within 30 days.** The hospital may respond within 30 days that it intends to submit an application to operate the unit as a provider-based unit or a freestanding (non-provider-based) entity. The hospital must then submit the appropriate application within 90 days.

  - **Application to operate as a freestanding entity.** The hospital may choose to submit an application to operate the department as a freestanding unit (e.g., certified ambulatory surgery center, independent diagnostic testing center, federally qualified health center, freestanding physician clinic). If this application is submitted within 90 days of the hospital's response, CMS will continue to pay the unit at the freestanding rate until a final determination is made about the hospital's application.

  - **Application to operate as a provider-based unit.** The hospital may choose to submit an application to operate the department as a provider-based unit. The hospital must submit an attestation with that application. If this application is submitted within 90 days of the hospital's response, CMS will pay the hospital on a temporary basis for services furnished in the unit at the higher provider-based rate until a final determination is made on the hospital's application. If the application is denied, CMS will recoup the higher amounts paid to the hospital during the application process.

  - **No application submitted.** If the hospital fails to submit the application within 90 days after the hospital's initial response, then CMS will stop all payments for services furnished in the unit.

- **Hospital fails to respond within 30 days.** If the hospital fails to respond within 30 days, CMS will:

    – Stop all payments for the unit at issue after 30 days.

    – Recoup all payments for the unit as discussed in the notice. Payments will be adjusted to reflect the amounts that would have been paid for the services as a freestanding facility.

Regardless of the actions taken by the hospital, CMS will recoup any payments made at the higher provider-based rate for all prior cost-reporting periods as described in the notice. Notably, if the entity had grandfathered status (see Chapter 3), recoupment will be limited to periods beginning after the grandfathering period—the start of the hospital's first cost-reporting period beginning on or after July 1, 2003 (42 *CFR* §413.65[b][2], 2011). In addition, recoupment is limited when a hospital has submitted an attestation regarding the provider-based department (*Transmittal A-03-030*, Section B.3, 2003). In that case, the recoupment starts only after the date the attestation was submitted, even if that is the same attestation that was denied, causing the recoupment to be incurred.

There is one other exception to this recoupment process, where the hospital has demonstrated a good faith effort to comply with the provider-based requirements but failed to meet every one of these requirements. In particular, CMS will limit the amount of the recoupment if the hospital complied with the following provider-based requirements:

1. The unit was included under the hospital licensure, as required under 42 *CFR* §413.65(d)(1) (2011)

2. There was signage and other information furnished to the public to ensure that the public was aware that the unit was a provider-based department, as detailed in 42 *CFR* §413.65(d)(4) (2011)

3. The facility services were billed as if they were furnished by a provider-based department

4. The professional services of the physicians and nonphysician practitioners were billed with the correct POS codes, as explained in 42 *CFR* §413.65(g)(2) (2011)

    —42 *CFR* §413.65(j)(2), 2011.

If the hospital demonstrated this good faith effort, CMS will not recoup any higher amounts paid for services before the beginning of the hospital's first cost-reporting period beginning on or after January 10, 2001 (42 *CFR* §413.65[j][2], 2011). This could be a significant savings in the recoupment process. Given this, hospitals should consider these to be the most essential of the list of provider-based requirements and should audit to ensure that all of their provider-based departments always meet at least these requirements.

A process flow chart for the audit response and recoupment process is included for your convenience (see Figure 4.2 at the end of this chapter).

In addition, the provider may request that CMS reconsider a determination that it does not qualify for provider-based status and may appeal an adverse reconsideration decision before an ALJ of the DAB under the provisions of 42 *CFR* Part 498 (2011). As described in *Transmittal A-03-030* (2003):

> *"Regardless of whether or how it responds to the notice in items (1) through (3) above, the provider may choose to appeal its denial of provider-based status within 60 days from the date of the notice of denial. Adverse determinations regarding provider-based status may be appealed under the administrative appeals procedures set forth in 42 CFR Part 498. Any notice to the provider of an adverse determination must contain a paragraph informing the provider of its right to appeal under those procedures. The following language may be used to inform the provider of its appeal rights:*
>
> *Initial Determination Request for Reconsideration*
> *If you are dissatisfied with this determination, you may request reconsideration by filing a written reconsideration request within sixty (60) days from the date on which you receive this letter. Your request must state the issues or findings of fact with which you disagree and the reasons for disagreement. Your reconsideration rights are set forth in the regulations at 42 CFR §498.22. Please address your request for reconsideration to:*
> *(Insert address of appropriate CMS RO ARA [Associate Regional Administrator].)*
>
> *Denial of a Reconsideration Request*
> *If you disagree with this first level appeals determination, you or your legal representative may request a hearing before an Administrative Law Judge (ALJ) of the Department of Health and Human Services, Departmental Appeals Board. Procedures governing this process are set out in the regulations at 42 CFR §498.40 et seq. A written request for a hearing must be filed within sixty (60) days from the date on which you receive your first level appeal results. The request should be made to:*
>
> *Departmental Appeals Board*
> *Civil Remedies Division*
> *Room 637-D*
> *Hubert H. Humphrey Building*
> *200 Independence Avenue, S.W.*
> *Washington, D.C. 20201*
> *Attention: Jacqueline Williams*

Forward a copy of your request for an ALJ hearing to:

(Insert address of appropriate CMS RO ARA.)

and

(Insert address of appropriate RO General Counsel.)

A request for a hearing must identify the specific issues and findings of fact and conclusions of law with which you disagree, and specify the basis for contending that the findings and conclusions are incorrect."

—Transmittal A-03-030, Section E.8(3), 2003.

Hospitals are allowed to simultaneously respond to the RO's denial by both applying for the provider-based status and appealing the denial to the DAB.

Self-disclosure of failure to comply with provider-based rules

Even if a hospital does not receive a notice from CMS, but has reason to believe that the provider-based requirements are not met for a department that the hospital is treating as a provider-based unit, the hospital is still required to take action. As described in previous chapters, hospitals generally receive a higher rate of reimbursement for provider-based departments as compared to freestanding entities. If the hospital learns that it failed to ensure that the provider-based requirements are met for the unit, and the hospital has received additional payments based on this status, this means that the hospital has knowledge of having received overpayments for the services furnished in that unit.

Medicare and Medicaid providers and suppliers have always had an obligation to refund overpayments from federal healthcare programs. However, Section 6402 of the Affordable Care Act (ACA) (42 *USC* §1320a–7k[d], 2010) creates liability under the Federal False Claims Act (31 *USC* §§3729–3733, 2011) for persons who fail to disclose and refund Medicare or Medicaid overpayments within the later of either 60 days after the date the overpayment is identified or the date the next applicable cost report is due. Section 6402 of the ACA is self-implementing. Therefore, all Medicare providers and suppliers have an obligation to report and refund overpayments within the time frame set out in the ACA statute. If the provider retains these funds with the knowledge that this constitutes an overpayment, this could be considered a violation of the False Claims Act, which is punishable by both criminal and civil penalties. As discussed above, the recent settlement agreements reached by Our Lady of Lourdes Memorial Hospital and Allegiance Health with the OIG and the United States Attorney's Office were based on the hospital's self-disclosure of noncompliance with the provider-based requirements.

Hospitals should consult with legal counsel if information comes to light that indicates that any hospital department has been billed as a provider-based entity without meeting the necessary requirements. Counsel may advise the hospital to self-disclose and repay the overpayment to avoid liability under the Federal False Claims Act.

Scenarios

The following scenarios will assist in understanding some of the complexities of attestations and provider-based determinations.

Scenario A

Hospital XYZ acquired an off-campus cardiology clinic 40 miles from the hospital campus on January 1, 2012, and started operating the location as a provider-based clinic. The patients are registered and billed by the hospital as hospital outpatients.

The hospital submitted an attestation to the RO and MAC for this clinic on January 1, 2013, requesting provider-based status. The RO sent a notice to the hospital dated January 1, 2014, denying provider-based status for this clinic. The RO explained that the clinic is located further than 35 miles from the main hospital campus and does not meet any of the other exceptions under 42 *CFR* §413.65(e) (2011) that would demonstrate that the clinic is integrated with the hospital. In addition, the RO reported that the physicians billing for services in this clinic have been using POS 11 on their professional claims.

The hospital decides to run this clinic as a freestanding physician office. The chief financial officer (CFO) calls you into his office and wants to know how far back the RO will recoup, how the recoupment calculation will be performed, and what correspondence has to be sent to the RO at this point.

Response:

As explained in *Transmittal A-03-030*, Section B.3 (2003), the recoupment for the denial of this attestation limits the recoupment to the period beginning after January 1, 2013, even though the hospital has technically been operating this clinic in violation of the provider-based requirements since January 1, 2012. The amount of the recoupment for that one-year period will be the amount paid to the hospital that exceeds the amount that would have been paid for a freestanding physician clinic.

The hospital is required to respond to the RO's notice within 30 days, stating that the clinic will be operated as a freestanding physician office. During that time, the services furnished there will be reimbursed at a freestanding rate. The hospital then must respond within another 90 days, submitting any paperwork necessary to formalize the use of the clinic as a freestanding clinic. If the hospital does not submit the required responses, all payments will be halted for these services.

As a side note, the hospital should be aware that the physicians may also be subject to recoupment of the payments that they received in excess of the MPFS amount that was due them for these services that were furnished in a facility rather than in a physician office setting.

© 2015 HCPro

Scenario B

Same scenario as above, except the hospital decides to operate the clinic as a provider-based clinic. The CFO wants to know what would be different in this case.

Response:

There would be no change in the recoupment amount and calculation. However, the hospital would be required to respond to the RO within 30 days that the intention is to operate the clinic as provider-based. If that is done timely, the services will be temporarily reimbursed at a *provider-based* rate. The hospital must then submit the application for provider-based status within 90 days, or all payments for the clinic will cease.

If the application is submitted timely, includes the attestation, and is complete, then provider-based payments will be continued until the application is approved or denied.

The hospital will be required to remediate the adverse findings made by the RO, including working with the physicians to correct the POS coding and moving the clinic closer to the hospital. Of course, the hospital should audit the clinic to ensure compliance with all other requirements.

Scenario C

Same scenario as above, but the hospital believes that the RO determination is incorrect and wants to appeal the determination. The CFO wants to know if this is possible.

Response:

The hospital may simultaneously respond to the RO's denial by applying for the provider-based status, as described in Scenario B, and appeal the denial to the DAB. In order to appeal the denial, the hospital must follow the appeal process described in 42 *CFR* Part 498 (2011). The first step in this appeal process is to file a request for hearing to the ALJ of the DAB within 60 days of the date of receipt of the denial notice.

Figure 4.1	Sample Attestation Format

SAMPLE ATTESTATION FORMAT

The following is an example of an acceptable format for an attestation of provider-based compliance.

Please note that provider-based determinations in relation to hospitals are not made for the following facilities: ambulatory surgical centers (ASCs), comprehensive outpatient rehabilitation facilities (CORFs), home health agencies (HHAs), skilled nursing facilities (SNFs), hospices, inpatient rehabilitation units that are excluded from the inpatient prospective payment system for acute hospital services, independent diagnostic testing facilities furnishing only services paid under a fee schedule (subject to §413.65(a)(1)(ii)(G)), facilities other than those operating as parts of CAHs that furnish only physical, occupational, or speech therapy to ambulatory patients (subject to § 413.65(a)(1)(ii)(H)), ESRD facilities, departments of providers that perform functions necessary for the successful operation of the providers but do not furnish services of a type for which separate payment could be claimed under Medicare or Medicaid (for example, laundry or medical records departments), ambulances.

(**Note:** As of the date of release of this Program Memorandum, legislation has not been enacted to further extend the moratorium on applying the $1,500 annual cap on physical therapy, occupational therapy, and speech therapy services of providers and suppliers other than hospitals).

Provider-Based Status Attestation Statement

Main provider's Medicare Provider Number:_____

Main provider's name:_____

Main provider's address:_____

Application contact name and phone number _____

Facility/Organization's name: _____

Facility/Organization's **exact** address:_____

    (Include bldg. no., suite/room no., etc.) _____

Facility/Organization's Medicare Provider Number, if there is one: _____

Is the facility/organization part of a multi-campus hospital? _____

Is the facility a Federally Qualified Health Center (FQHC)? If so, and if the FQHC meets the criteria at section 413.65(n), it need not attest to its provider-based status. The provider-based rules do not apply to other FQHCs that do not meet the criteria at section 413.65(n), and an attestation should not be submitted.

The facility/organization became provider-based with the main provider on the following date:_____

(Please indicate if this attestation is adding deleting, or changing previous information—if yes, please make certain to include the effective date.)

Figure 4.1	Sample Attestation Format (cont.)

Indicate whether the facility/organization is "on campus" or "off campus" (per § 413.65(a)(2)) with the main provider:

1. _____ **On campus** of the main provider (located within 250 yards from the main provider building)

OR

2. _____ **Off campus** of the main provider (located 250 yards or greater from the main provider building, but subject to § 413.65(e)(3))

I certify that I have carefully read the attached sections of the Federal provider-based regulations, before signing this attestation, and that the facility/organization complies with the following requirements to be provider-based to the main provider (initial ONE selection only):

1. _____ The facility/organization is "**on campus**" per 42 *CFR* §413.65(a)(2) and is in compliance with the following provider-based requirements (shown in the following attached pages) in §413.65(d) and §413.65(g), other than those in §413.65(g)(7). If the facility/organization is operated as a joint venture, I certify that the requirements under §413.65(f) have been met. I am aware of, and will comply with, the requirement to maintain documentation of the basis for these attestations (for each regulatory requirement) and to make that documentation available to the Centers for Medicare & Medicaid Services (CMS) and to CMS contractors upon request.

OR

2. _____ The facility/organization is "**off campus**" per 42 *CFR* §413.65(a)(2) and is in compliance with the following provider-based requirements (shown in the following attached pages) in §413.65(d) and §413.65(e) and §413.65(g). If the facility/organization is operated under a management contract/agreement, I certify that the requirements of §413.65(h) have been met. Furthermore, I am submitting, along with this attestation to the Centers for Medicare & Medicaid Services (CMS), the documentation showing the basis for these attestations (for each regulatory requirement).

Please complete the following for on-campus AND off-campus facilities and organizations:

I attest that the facility/organization complies with the following requirements to be provider-based to the main provider (please indicate Yes or No for each requirement):

1. _____ The department of the provider, the remote location of a hospital, or the satellite facility and the main provider are operated under the same license, except in areas where the State requires a separate license for the department of the provider, the remote location of a hospital, or the satellite facility, or in states where state law does not permit licensure of the provider and the prospective department of the provider, the remote location of a hospital, or the satellite facility under a single license. If the provider and facility/organization are located in a state having a health facilities' cost review commission or other agency that has authority to regulate the rates charged by hospitals or other providers, the commission or agency has not found that the facility/organization is not part of the provider.

2. _____ The clinical services of the facility or organization seeking provider-based status and the main provider are integrated.

Figure 4.1	Sample Attestation Format (cont.)

2a. _____ Professional staff of the facility or organization have clinical privileges at the main provider.

2b. _____ The main provider maintains the same monitoring and oversight of the facility or organization as it does for any other department of the provider.

2c. _____ The medical director of the facility or organization seeking provider-based status maintains a reporting relationship with the chief medical officer or other similar official of the main provider that has the same frequency, intensity, and level of accountability that exists in the relationship between the medical director of a department of the main provider and the chief medical officer or other similar official of the main provider, and is under the same type of supervision and accountability as any other director, medical or otherwise, of the main provider.

2d. _____ Medical staff committees or other professional committees at the main provider are responsible for medical activities in the facility or organization, including quality assurance, utilization review, and the coordination and integration of services, to the extent practicable, between the facility or organization seeking provider-based status and the main provider.

2e. _____ Medical records for patients treated in the facility or organization are integrated into a unified retrieval system (or cross reference) of the main provider.

2f. _____ Inpatient and outpatient services of the facility or organization and the main provider are integrated, and patients treated at the facility or organization who require further care have full access to all services of the main provider and are referred where appropriate to the corresponding inpatient or outpatient department or service of the main provider.

3. _____ The financial operations of the facility or organization are fully integrated within the financial system of the main provider, as evidenced by shared income and expenses between the main provider and the facility or organization. The costs of a facility or organization that is a hospital department are reported in a cost center of the provider; costs of a provider-based facility or organization other than a hospital department are reported in the appropriate cost center or cost centers of the main provider; and the financial status of any provider-based facility or organization is incorporated and readily identified in the main provider's trial balance.

4. _____ The facility or organization seeking status as a department of a provider, a remote location of a hospital, or a satellite facility is held out to the public and other payers as part of the main provider. When patients enter the provider-based facility or organization, they are aware that they are entering the main provider and are billed accordingly.

5. _____ In the case of a hospital outpatient department or a hospital-based entity (**if the facility is not a hospital outpatient department or a hospital-based entity, please record "NA" for "not applicable" and skip to requirements under number 6)**, the facility or organization fulfills the obligation of:

5a. _____ Hospital outpatient departments located either on or off the campus of the hospital that is the main provider comply with the anti-dumping rules in §§489.20(l), (m), (q), and (r) and §489.24 of chapter IV of Title 42.

 © 2015 HCPro

Figure 4.1	Sample Attestation Format (cont.)

5b. _____ Physician services furnished in hospital outpatient departments or hospital-based entities (other than RHCs) are billed with the correct site-of-service so that appropriate physician and practitioner payment amounts can be determined under the rules of Part 414 of chapter IV of Title 42.

5c. _____ Hospital outpatient departments comply with all the terms of the hospital's provider agreement.

5d. _____ Physicians who work in hospital outpatient departments or hospital-based entities comply with the non-discrimination provisions in §489.10(b) of chapter IV of Title 42.

5e. _____ Hospital outpatient departments (other than RHCs) treat all Medicare patients, for billing purposes, as hospital outpatients. The departments do not treat some Medicare patients as hospital outpatients and others as physician office patients.

5f. _____ In the case of a patient admitted to the hospital as an inpatient after receiving treatment in the hospital outpatient department or hospital-based entity, payments for services in the hospital outpatient department or hospital-based entity are subject to the payment window provisions applicable to PPS hospitals and to hospitals and units excluded from PPS set forth at §412.2(c)(5) of chapter IV of Title 42 and at § 413.40(c)(2) of chapter IV of Title 42, respectively. **(Note: If the potential main provider is a CAH, enter "NA" for this item.)**

5g. _____ **(Note: This requirement only applies to off campus facilities).** When a Medicare beneficiary is treated in a hospital outpatient department or hospital-based entity (other than an RHC) that is not located on the main provider's campus, and the treatment is not required to be provided by the antidumping rules in §489.24 of chapter IV of Title 42, the hospital provides written notice to the beneficiary, before the delivery of services, of the amount of the beneficiary's potential financial liability (that is, that the beneficiary will incur a coinsurance liability for an outpatient visit to the hospital as well as for the physician service, and of the amount of that liability).

(1) _____ The notice is one that the beneficiary can read and understand.

(2) _____ If the exact type and extent of care needed is not known, the hospital furnishes a written notice to the patient that explains that the beneficiary will incur a coinsurance liability to the hospital that he or she would not incur if the facility were not provider-based.

(3) _____ The hospital furnishes an estimate based on typical or average charges for visits to the facility, but states that the patient's actual liability will depend upon the actual services furnished by the hospital.

(4) _____ If the beneficiary is unconscious, under great duress, or for any other reason is unable to read a written notice and understand and act on his or her own rights, the notice is provided before the delivery of services to the beneficiary's authorized representative.

Figure 4.1	Sample Attestation Format (cont.)

(5) _____ In cases where a hospital outpatient department provides examination or treatment that is required to be provided by the anti-dumping rules at §489.24 of chapter IV of Title 42, the notice is given as soon as possible after the existence of an emergency condition has been ruled out or the emergency condition has been stabilized.

5h. _____ Hospital outpatient departments meet applicable hospital health and safety rules for Medicare-participating hospitals in part 482 of this chapter.

For off-campus facilities, please complete the following:

In addition to the above requirements (numbers 1–5h), I attest that the facility/organization complies with the following requirements to be provider-based to the main provider as an off-campus facility (please indicate Yes or No for each requirement):

6. _____ The facility or organization seeking provider-based status is operated under the ownership and control of the main provider, as evidenced by the following:

6a. _____ The business enterprise that constitutes the facility or organization is 100% owned by the provider.

6b. _____ The main provider and the facility or organization seeking status as a department of the provider, a remote location of a hospital, or a satellite facility have the same governing body.

6c. _____ The facility or organization is operated under the same organizational documents as the main provider. For example, the facility or organization seeking provider-based status is subject to common bylaws and operating decisions of the governing body of the provider where it is based.

6d. _____ The main provider has final responsibility for administrative decisions, final approval for contracts with outside parties, final approval for personnel actions, final responsibility for personnel policies (such as fringe benefits or code of conduct), and final approval for medical staff appointments in the facility or organization.

7. _____ The reporting relationship between the facility or organization seeking provider-based status and the main provider has the same frequency, intensity, and level of accountability that exists in the relationship between the main provider and one of its existing departments, as evidenced by compliance with all of the following requirements:

7a. _____ The facility or organization is under the direct supervision of the main provider.

7b. _____ The facility or organization is operated under the same monitoring and oversightby the provider as any other department of the provider, and is operated just as any other department of the provider with regard to supervision and accountability. The facility or organization director or individual responsible for daily operations at the entity

(1) _____ Maintains a reporting relationship with a manager at the main provider that has the same frequency, intensity, and level of accountability that exists in the relationship between the main provider and its existing departments; and

© 2015 HCPro

Figure 4.1	Sample Attestation Format (cont.)

      (2) _____ Is accountable to the governing body of the main provider, in the same manner as any department head of the provider.

7c. _____ The following administrative functions of the facility or organization are integrated with those of the provider where the facility or organization is based: billing services, records, human resources, payroll, employee benefit package, salary structure, and purchasing services. Either the same employees or group of employees handle these administrative functions for the facility or organization and the main provider, or the administrative functions for both the facility or organization and the entity are (1) contracted out under the same contract agreement; or (2) handled under different contract agreements, with the contract of the facility or organization being managed by the main provider.

8. The facility or organization is located within a 35-mile radius of the campus of the potential main provider, except when the requirements in paragraph 8a of this section are met (please check below in the appropriate location if you qualify for the exemption):

8a. _____ The facility or organization is owned and operated by a hospital or CAH that has a disproportionate share adjustment (as determined under §412.106 of chapter IV of Title 42) greater than 11.75% or is described in §412.106(c)(2) of chapter IV of Title 42 implementing section 1886(e)(5)(F)(i)(II) of the Act and is:

      (1) _____ Owned or operated by a unit of State or local government;

      (2) _____ A public or nonprofit corporation that is formally granted governmental powers by a unit of State or local government; or

      (3) _____ A private hospital that has a contract with a State or local government that includes the operation of clinics located off the main campus of the hospital to ensure access in a well-defined service area to healthcare services for low-income individuals who are not entitled to benefits under Medicare (or medical assistance under a Medicaid State plan).

8b. _____ The facility or organization demonstrates a high level of integration with the main provider by showing that it meets all of the other provider-based criteria and demonstrates that it serves the same patient population as the main provider, by submitting records showing that, during the 12-month period immediately preceding the first day of the month in which the attestation for provider-based status is filed with CMS, and for each subsequent 12-month period:

      (1) _____ At least 75% of the patients served by the facility or organization reside in the same Zip code areas as at least 75% of the patients served by the main provider;

      (2) _____ At least 75% of the patients served by the facility or organization who required the type of care furnished by the main provider received that care from that provider (for example, at least 75% of the patients of an RHC seeking provider-based status received inpatient hospital services from the hospital that is the main provider); or

Figure 4.1	Sample Attestation Format (cont.)

(3) _____ If the facility or organization is unable to meet the criteria in (1) or (2) directly above because it was not in operation during all of the 12-month period described in paragraph 8b, the facility or organization is located in a Zip code area included among those that, during all of the 12-month period described in paragraph 8b, accounted for at least 75% of the patients served by the main provider.

8c. _____ If the facility or organization is attempting to qualify for provider-based status under this section, then the facility or organization and the main provider are located in the same State or, when consistent with the laws of both States, in adjacent States.

Note: An RHC that is otherwise qualified as a provider-based entity of a hospital that is located in a rural area as defined in §412.62(f)(1)(iii) of chapter IV of Title 42, and has fewer than 50 beds as determined under §412.105(b) of chapter IV of Title 42, is not subject to the criteria in 8a and 8b above.

9. _____ The facility or organization that is not located on the campus of the potential main provider and otherwise meets the requirements of 1–8 above, but is operated under management contract, meets all of the following criteria (**please respond to 9a–9d if the facility is operated under a management contract; otherwise record "NA" for "not applicable"**):

9a. _____ The main provider (or an organization that also employs the staff of the main provider and that is not the management company) employs the staff of the facility or organization who are directly involved in the delivery of patient care, except for management staff and staff who furnish patient care services of a type that would be paid for by Medicare under a fee schedule established by regulations at Part 414 of chapter IV of Title 42. Other than staff that may be paid under such a Medicare fee schedule, the main provider does not utilize the services of "leased" employees (that is, personnel who are actually employed by the management company but provide services for the provider under a staff leasing or similar agreement) that are directly involved in the delivery of patient care.

9b. _____ The administrative functions of the facility or organization are integrated with those of the main provider, as determined under criteria in paragraph 7c above.

9c. _____ The main provider has significant control over the operations of the facility or organization as determined under criteria in paragraph 7b above.

9d. _____ The management contract is held by the main provider itself, not by a parent organization that has control over both the main provider and the facility or organization.

For facilities/organizations operated as joint ventures requesting provider-based determinations: In addition to the above requirements (numbers 1–5h for on campus facilities), I attest

Figure 4.1	Sample Attestation Format (cont.)

that the facility/organization complies with the following requirements to be provider-based to the main provider:

10. _____ The facility or organization being attested to as provider-based is a joint venture that fulfills the following requirements:

10a. _____ The facility is partially owned by at least one provider;

10b. _____ The facility is located on the main campus of a provider who is a partial owner;

10c. _____ The facility is provider-based to that one provider whose campus on which the facility organization is located; and

10d. _____ The facility or organization meets all the requirements applicable to all provider-based facilities and organizations in paragraphs 1–5 of this attestation.

* I certify that the responses in this attestation and information in the documents are accurate, complete, and current as of this date. I acknowledge that the regulations must be continually adhered to. Any material change in the relationship between the facility/organization and the main provider, such as a change of ownership or entry into a new or different management contract, may be reported to CMS. (NOTE: ORIGINAL ink signature must be submitted)

Signed: _____

(Signature of Officer or Administrator or authorized person)

_____

(PRINT Name of signature)

Title: _____

(Title of authorized person acting on behalf of the provider)

_____

(Direct telephone number)

Date: _____

* Whoever, in any matter within the jurisdiction of any department or agency of the United States knowingly and willfully falsifies, conceals, or covers up by any trick, scheme, or device a material fact, or makes any false, fictitious, or fraudulent statement or representations, or makes or uses any false writing or document knowing the same to contain any false, fictitious, or fraudulent statement or entry, shall be fined not more than $10,000 or imprisoned not more than five years or both. (18 *USC* § 1001).

Source: Transmittal A-03-030 - Provider-Based Status On or After October 1, 2002. *(2003.) Retrieved May 22, 2015, from www.cms. gov/Regulations-and-Guidance/Guidance/Transmittals/downloads/A03030.pdf.*

Figure 4.2 Response Summary When a Provider Fails an Audit

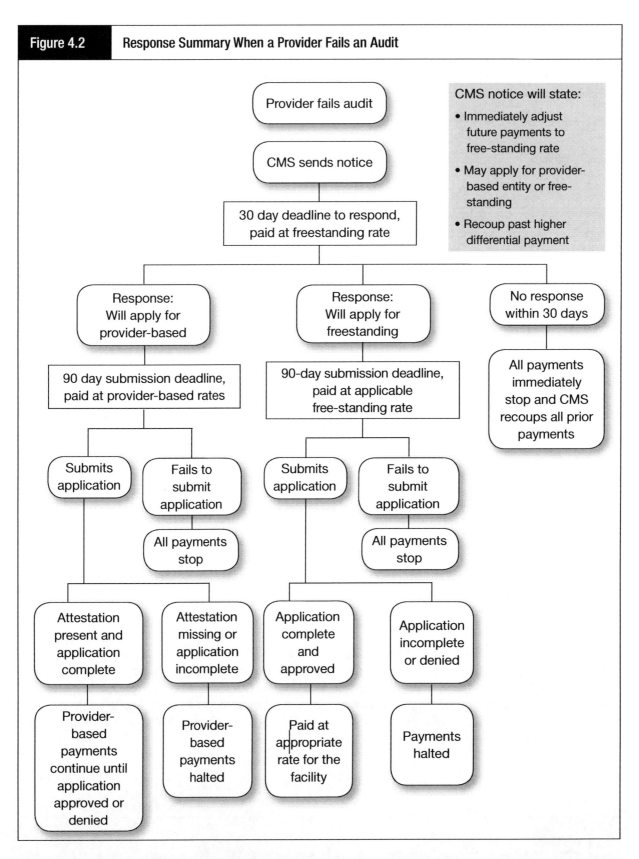

*Source: **Gina M. Reese, Esq., RN,** an instructor for HCPro's Medicare Boot Camp®—Hospital Version and Medicare Boot Camp®—Utilization Review Version. Reprinted with permission.*

© 2015 HCPro

Medicare Coverage of Outpatient Hospital Services Furnished in Provider-Based Departments

Overview

As discussed in previous chapters, in order to qualify as a provider-based department, the hospital must treat the location just like any other hospital outpatient department. We have covered some of those requirements in some detail in Chapter 3. In that discussion, we referenced in general that the hospital must comply with Medicare *CoPs*, coverage, and payment rules. This includes, among other things, ensuring that the services furnished in a provider-based department meet the coverage rules for services furnished to Medicare beneficiaries in hospital outpatient departments (42 *CFR* 413.65[g][3], 2011).

There are three main types of services furnished in a hospital outpatient department—therapeutic, diagnostic, and drugs—which each have their own coverage requirements. These coverage rules dictate, among other things, that outpatient therapeutic and diagnostic services be ordered, supervised, and overseen in a specified fashion.

Coverage of Hospital Outpatient Therapeutic Services

One of the most basic of the Medicare coverage rules is the requirement that therapeutic services paid under the hospital OPPS, or paid on a reasonable cost basis to CAHs, must be furnished "incident to" a physician's services (42 *CFR* §410.27, 2011). As hospital outpatient departments, services furnished in provider-based departments must also meet these coverage requirements (42 *CFR* §413.65, 2011).

Notably, certain services furnished in OPPS hospitals are not paid by Medicare under OPPS. Instead, these services are paid under a payment scheme designed specifically for them. As a consequence, these services are not subject to the "incident to" coverage rules (76 *Fed. Reg.* 74122, 74369–70, 2011). For example, PT, OT, and SLP services are not subject to these rules, because they are excluded from payment under OPPS. Instead, these services are paid under the MPFS and are subject to a different set of coverage rules (*Medicare Claims Processing Manual*, Chapter 5, §§10.2, 10.4, 20, 2015; 42 *CFR* §§410.59, 410.60, 410.62, 2011).

Other services that are excluded from payment under OPPS, and therefore also exempt from the general Medicare coverage rules for therapeutic services, include:

- Annual wellness visits (42 *CFR* §410.15, 2011)
- Initial preventive physical examination (42 *CFR* §410.16, 2011)
- Medical supplies, appliances, and devices (42 *CFR* §410.36, 2011)
- Durable medical equipment (42 *CFR* §410.38, 2010)
- Ambulance services (42 *CFR* §410.40, 2010)
- Partial hospitalization services (42 *CFR* §410.43, 2011)
- Pulmonary rehabilitation program (42 *CFR* §410.47, 2010)
- Kidney disease education services (42 *CFR* §410.48, 2011)
- Cardiac rehabilitation program and intensive cardiac rehabilitation program (42 *CFR* §410.49, 2009)
- Dialysis services and supplies (42 *CFR* §410.50, 2011)
- Pneumococcal vaccine and flu vaccine (42 *CFR* §410.57, 2011)
- Hepatitis B vaccine and blood clotting factors (42 *CFR* §410.63, 2011)
- Telehealth services (42 *CFR* §410.78, 2011)

These services do have their own Medicare coverage requirements, which may be stricter or less onerous than the general coverage rules for therapeutic services. Hospitals must review these separate requirements for each of these services to ensure that these rules are followed in provider-based departments.

A handful of other services are also excluded from these requirements, because there are also separate Medicare coverage rules for those services. For example, drugs furnished to hospital outpatients are covered under a separate category by Medicare and have their own coverage requirements (*Medicare Benefit Policy Manual*, Chapter 15 §50 et seq., 2014).

What are therapeutic services?

Therapeutic services include most non-diagnostic services furnished to patients in clinics, emergency departments, and urgent care centers to treat, rather than diagnose, the patient's condition. These include patient examinations and assessments, surgical services, and minor procedures such as wound care, medication management, and infusions (42 *CFR* §410.27[a], 2011; *Medicare Benefit Policy Manual*, Chapter 6, §20.5.1, 2014). Diagnostic services such as x-rays, electroencephalograms, electrocardiograms, and laboratory tests have separate coverage requirements and will be discussed below.

Note that we are referring here to the facility component of the therapeutic services furnished to Medicare beneficiaries, which is furnished by the hospital (including provider-based departments). We are not including in this discussion the professional services furnished to the patient by physicians and other nonphysician practitioners (NPP) who bill separately for these services. Payment for facility services is separate and distinct from payment for professional services, as discussed in detail in Chapter 6. Therefore, do not make the mistake of confusing the facility component of therapeutic services with the professional component of these services when reviewing the Medicare "incident to" rules discussed below.

Compliance with the "incident to" rules

There are four main requirements that must be met for a service to meet the "incident to" rules. These rules are spelled out in 42 *CFR* §410.27 (2011) and the *Medicare Benefit Policy Manual*, Chapter 6, §20.5.1 (2014). In order to qualify, the service must be:

- Furnished directly by the hospital or under arrangements by the hospital and in the hospital or a provider-based department of the hospital (42 *CFR* §§410.27[a][1][i], [iii], 2011; *Medicare Benefit Policy Manual*, Chapter 6, §20.5.2, 2014)

- Furnished on the order of a physician or NPP working within their scope of practice (*Medicare Benefit Policy Manual*, Chapter 6, §20.5.2, 2014)

- Furnished as an integral, although incidental, part of a physician or nonphysician services in the course of diagnosing or treating the patient (42 *CFR* §§410.27[a][1][ii], 2011; *Medicare Benefit Policy Manual*, Chapter 6, §20.5.2, 2014)

- Furnished under the appropriate level of supervision by a physician or nonphysician practitioner (42 *CFR* §§410.27[a][1][iv], 2011)

Some of these requirements are fairly straightforward and intuitively easy to meet, while others are more complex. It is essential, however, that hospital leadership completely understand these requirements. Failure to meet any component of these rules means that a service is not covered by Medicare *at all* and that any payment received by the hospital for the service may be considered an overpayment.

Furnished by the Hospital Directly or Under Arrangements

The requirement that outpatient services must be furnished by the hospital directly or under arrangements is fairly self-explanatory, but may be tricky in some situations. The basic idea is that a hospital cannot bill Medicare for a hospital outpatient service unless that hospital actually furnishes the services. If another facility is actually furnishing the services without hospital oversight or control, the patient may not be considered a hospital outpatient, and the hospital should not be billing for that service.

The hospital usually furnishes the services directly, which means that the service is provided by the hospital's own employees. However, in lieu of using its own employees, the hospital may contract with another entity to furnish the service under arrangements using that other company's employees and, at times, in the facility of the other entity.

When the hospital furnishes the services directly, it must do so within the hospital itself or in a provider-based department. The trick is that the provider-based department that furnishes the services must actually completely meet the provider-based requirements. If, for some reason, the hospital fails to ensure that the rules are not met for the provider-based department, then the Medicare "incident to" rules are not met, and the services may considered to be non-covered. In that case, the unit where the services were furnished would be treated as a freestanding clinic, and the hospital would have no authority to bill Medicare for the services furnished there.

Order of a Physician or Nonphysician Practitioner

Under the "incident to" rules, the services furnished to a hospital outpatient may be performed only under the order of a physician or NPP working within his or her scope of practice (*Medicare Benefit Policy Manual*, Chapter 6, §20.5.2, 2014). This is referred to herein as the "physician order rule." It is likely that hospital leadership assumes that all services are furnished only under a physician's order and, therefore, that this requirement is simple to meet. Surprisingly, this is not always the case, and, hence, this requirement should be audited periodically.

It is not sufficient that just any physician or NPP order the services. The physician or NPP may only order services that are within his or her scope of practice (*Medicare Benefit Policy Manual*, Chapter 6, §20.5.2, 2014). This is more of an issue with NPPs, whose scope of practice is generally more limited than that of physicians. In addition, in accordance with Medicare *CoP*s, the physician or NPP ordering the services must have clinical privileges at the hospital, and the services ordered by the physician or NPP must lie within the scope of those clinical privileges. While this seems obvious, it is another point that should be audited.

Integral, Although Incidental, Part of Physician's Service

CMS requires that hospital outpatient services be furnished as an integral, although incidental, part of the physician services. This requirement is related to the physician order rule discussed above and has many of the same pitfalls. Under this rule, the physician must see a patient periodically and sufficiently often enough to assess the course of the patient's treatment and the patient's progress, and, where necessary, to change the treatment regimen (*Medicare Benefit Policy Manual*, Chapter 6, §20.5.2, 2011). The physician is not required to see the patient each visit. In fact, as long as the physician writes an order for the services, and the services are properly supervised as detailed below, the nurses and other staff members may perform services over a significant period of time without the treating physician's personal presence in the clinic. This is quite common in the monitoring and treatment of chronic conditions, such as in diabetes, hypertension, anticoagulation, and wound care clinics.

However, it is not sufficient to just write an order and refer the patient to a hospital outpatient department without any further follow-up during the course of treatment (*Medicare Benefit Policy Manual*, Chapter 6, §20.5.2, 2014). For the services to be covered by Medicare, the hospital must demonstrate that the physician personally sees the patient periodically to assess the course of treatment and the patient's response to the treatment, and to change the treatment if the patient is not responding sufficiently to it. It is not sufficient for the nursing staff to simply call or otherwise communicate with the physician about the patient's condition. Instead, CMS intends for the physician's contact with the patient to be hands on to ensure that the physician personally examines the patient's condition.

Inherent in this requirement, as well as the companion requirement for a physician's order to initiate treatment, is the necessity for the physician to personally see and examine the patient at least once prior to the nurses initiating the treatment. Based on this rule, CMS has specifically mandated that services furnished to patients who leave a hospital outpatient department (including an emergency department) without seeing the physician are not Medicare-covered services (CMS Frequently Asked Questions 2297, n.d.). In that case, the hospital should not bill Medicare for even a low-level emergency department or clinic visit for those services, since they would not be in compliance with the "incident-to" rules. This is true even if the nurses are working under some type of standardized protocol that is otherwise allowed under their state scope of practice.

CMS does not specifically dictate the frequency of the physician's personal involvement. The frequency of the physician's visits with the patient after the initiation of the treatment would vary depending on the patient's condition, the type of treatment, and the patient's personal response to the treatment. For some rapidly changing conditions and unstable patients, the physician might need to see the patient frequently—even daily, several times a week, or more frequently, as necessary. For other more stable situations, the nursing staff may be able to monitor the patients for longer periods of time without physician involvement. However, even in those situations, it would not be reasonable to allow the physician's visits to be too sporadic. Even more stable patients should be examined by the physician at some minimum frequency (i.e., quarterly) during long periods of treatment. Hospitals may want to work with its medical staff to establish criteria for the frequency of physician visits for specific patients and conditions to aide in auditing this requirement.

If services are billed to Medicare without meeting any component of these rules, any payment received by the hospital could be considered an overpayment.

Appropriate Supervision of the Services by a Physician or Nonphysician Practitioner

Who may supervise the services

Prior to 2010, CMS only allowed physicians and clinical psychologists to act as supervisors for hospital outpatient services. However, in recognition of the difficulty in finding a sufficient number of physicians to act as supervisors for these services, CMS allowed NPPs to act as supervisors with specific limitations, effective January 1, 2010 (42 *CFR* 410.27[a][1], 2011; *Medicare Benefit Policy Manual*, Chapter 6, §20.5.2, 2014).

For purposes of this rule, NPPs include nurse practitioners, physician assistants, clinical nurse specialists, certified nurse midwives, clinical psychologists, and licensed clinical social workers (42 *CFR* 410.27[g], 2011; *Medicare Benefit Policy Manual*, Chapter 6 §20.5, 2014). Notably, this does not include certified registered nurse anesthetists; therefore, CRNAs may not act as supervisors of hospital outpatient services to meet the "incident to" requirements.

NPPs may only supervise services they are allowed to personally perform under their state scope of practice (*Medicare Benefit Policy Manual*, Chapter 6, §20.5.2, 2014). In addition, NPPs may not supervise cardiac, intensive cardiac, or pulmonary rehab service, because the Medicare regulations specifically mandate that these services be supervised by physicians (42 *CFR* 410.27[a][1][iv][D], 2011).

Supervision levels

CMS has defined three levels of supervision for different types of services. To understand the level of supervision necessary to comply with the "incident to" rules for hospital outpatient services, one must first understand the requirements for these levels of supervision, including:

- **General supervision.** General supervision is the most liberal type of supervision. CMS defines general supervision in 42 *CFR* §410.32(b)(3)(i) (2011), which requires that the services be furnished under the overall supervision and control of a physician, but does not require the physician to be personally present during the provision of the services (42 *CFR* §410.27[a][1][iv][B], 2011). Under this level of supervision, the physician effectively acts as the medical director for the hospital outpatient department. The medical director writes policies and procedures for the unit, monitors and oversees the quality of care furnished in the department, and is responsible for the clinical standards of care. Services in the department are still subject to the physician ordering rule and the requirement that the physician periodically see the patient in person to assess the effectiveness of the treatment, but there is no requirement that a physician or NPP remain in the department or be immediately available on a day-to-day basis.

- **Direct supervision.** When CMS requires that a service be furnished under direct supervision, the physician or NPP must be immediately available to furnish assistance and direction throughout the performance of the entire procedure (42 *CFR* §410.27[a][1][iv], 2011; *Medicare Benefit Policy Manual*, Chapter 6, §20.5.2, 2014). This does not mean that the physician or NPP must be present in the room when the procedure is performed. However, the supervising physician or NPP must meet the following requirements:

    - The supervising physician or NPP must be immediately available (42 *CFR* 410.27[a][1][iv], 2011; *Medicare Benefit Policy Manual*, Chapter 6, §20.5.2, 2014). According to CMS, this means that the physician is physically present and interruptible, is able to respond without lapse of time, and cannot be so physically distant that he or she is unable to intervene right away. The physician or NPP would not be considered to be available if he or she is occupied by a procedure or service that could not be interrupted, or if he or she is not able to step in and perform the service being supervised, if necessary (*Medicare Benefit Policy Manual*, Chapter 6, §20.5.2, 2014).

    - The physician or NPP must be able to furnish assistance and direction for the procedure he or she is supervising (*Medicare Benefit Policy Manual*, Chapter 6 §20.5, 2014). As part of this requirement, CMS mandates that the service the physician or NPP is supervising must be one he or she is allowed to perform within his or her scope of practice and hospital privileges. In addition, the physician or NPP must be able to step in and take over the provision of the procedure, not just respond to emergencies. This does not mean that the physician must be in the same specialty as the service being furnished, but he or she must be knowledgeable enough to take over the procedure and change the procedure or course of treatment for the patient, if necessary (*Medicare Benefit Policy Manual*, Chapter 6 §20.5, 2014).

The physician or NPP must be available throughout the performance of the procedure (*Medicare Benefit Policy Manual*, Chapter 6 §20.5, 2014).

- **Personal supervision.** Personal supervision is the easiest level of supervision to understand. If a service requires personal supervision, the physician or NPP must personally be present in the room for the duration of the entire procedure (42 *CFR* §410.2[a][1][iv][B], 2004; 42 *CFR* §410.32[b][3][iii], 2011). Personal supervision is not pertinent to the coverage requirements for therapeutic services, but is applicable to certain diagnostic services, as discussed further below.

Level of Supervision Required for Most Therapeutic Services in Hospital Outpatient Departments

Now that we have described CMS' three levels of supervision—general, direct, and personal—the next topic of discussion is which level of supervision applies to therapeutic services furnished in hospital outpatient departments. The answer is not that straightforward. Like with many Medicare regulations, the level of supervision depends on the particular service furnished along with other factors.

Prior to January 1, 2011, CMS required that all hospital outpatient services be furnished under a direct level of supervision, regardless of the location of the provider-based department (on-campus versus off-campus) (*Medicare Benefit Policy Manual*, Chapter 6 §20.5.2, 2014). This requirement was considered to be very onerous for many hospitals, especially CAHs and other hospitals in physician shortage areas, where it was already difficult to recruit sufficient numbers of physicians just to furnish basic medical services.

In response, CMS loosened these restrictions and created a new paradigm for the required level of supervision effective January 1, 2011. Under this new scheme, the default level of supervision for hospital outpatient services is direct supervision (42 *CFR* §410.27[a][1][iv], 2011; *Medicare Benefit Policy Manual*, Chapter 6 §20.5.2, 2014). However, as urged by hospitals nationwide, CMS conceded that some services which are relatively routine and low-risk may be furnished under general supervision. This takes two forms:

- Services that may be furnished under general supervision for all patients

- Nonsurgical extended duration therapeutic services (NSEDTS) that must be initiated under direct supervision and then may be allowed to move to general supervision for individual patients if the physician determines that the patient is stable

Therapeutic services that may be furnished under general supervision

CMS has set up a sub-regulatory process to review which services should be considered for designation as appropriate for general supervision for all patients based on recommendations from a Hospital Outpatient Payment Panel and comments from the hospital industry (76 *Fed. Reg.* 74122, 74370–71, 2011; *Medicare Benefit Policy Manual,* Chapter 6 §20.5.2, 2014). Under this process, hospitals and others in the hospital industry may request that the Hospital Outpatient Payment Panel review a particular service and recommend to CMS that it be approved to be provided under general supervision. The Panel meets twice a year (March and August) and considers the requests as they arrive based on the volume and cost of reimbursement for the service, as well as the frequency of requests for that service.

The Panel's preliminary decisions are posted for public comment for 30 days, and the final decisions are posted in July and January of each year. CMS publishes the list and effective date of these services on the OPPS home page of its website under "Hospital Outpatient Therapeutic Services That Have Been Evaluated for a Change in Supervision Level" (2015). A number of services have been added to this list over the years. For example, CMS approved 36592 (collect blood from peripherally inserted central catheter [PICC]) to be furnished under general supervision effective January 1, 2013, and approved the addition of 94668 (chest wall manipulation) to be furnished under general supervision effective July 1, 2014.

Nonsurgical extended duration therapeutic services

CMS made another concession in the recent regulations that recognized that while certain services are not always safe and effective and, therefore, do not qualify for general supervision per se, these services may be relatively safe for individual patients after they are stabilized on the treatment. CMS refers to these services as a "Nonsurgical Extended Duration Therapeutic Service" or "NSEDTS" (42 *CFR* §410.27[a][1][iv][E], 2011; *Medicare Benefit Policy Manual,* Chapter 6, §§20.5.2, 20.7, 2014). CMS mandates that NSEDTS services be initiated for all patients at a direct level of supervision. If and when the supervising physician determines that the individual patient is stable, then the remainder of the course of the treatment may be delivered under a general level of supervision. The supervising physician must document in the medical record for that specific patient that the patient is stable and that the NSEDTS service may safely transition from direct to general supervision (42 *CFR* §410.27[a][1][iv][E], 2011; *Medicare Benefit Policy Manual,* Chapter 6, §§20.5.2, 20.7, 2014).

In the implementing regulations, CMS defined a beginning set of these services. Similar to the list of services that may be furnished under general supervision, CMS publishes the list and effective date of the NSEDTS services on the OPPS home page of its website, under "Hospital Outpatient Therapeutic Services That Have Been Evaluated for a Change in Supervision Level" (2015). Just like for the general supervision level services, hospitals may petition to have other services added to the NSEDTS list through the sub-regulatory process described above. In fact, numerous services have been added to this list since its initiation. For example, C8957 (prolonged IV infusion requiring pump) was on the original list approved by CMS to be furnished as an NSEDTS service, and CMS approved G0379 (direct referral hospital observation) as a NSEDTS service effective January 1, 2013.

Remember that if the service does not appear on the CMS list, "Hospital Outpatient Therapeutic Services That Have Been Evaluated for a Change in Supervision Level," the service must be furnished under a direct level of supervision at all times. Failure to follow the dictated level of supervision may result in a finding that the reimbursement for the services was received erroneously and that the overpayments must be repaid.

Location of supervising physician

Prior to 2011, the supervising physician or NPP was required to remain on the hospital campus to supervise on-campus departments and in the actual outpatient department to supervise off-campus departments (*Medicare Benefit Policy Manual*, Chapter 6, §§20.5.2, 20.7, 2014). Along with the level of supervision requirement, this was an additional burden for many hospitals, especially CAHs and other hospitals in physician shortage areas, where it was already difficult to recruit sufficient numbers of physicians just to furnish basic medical services. Limiting the movement of the scarce number of physicians to the hospital outpatient departments or hospital campus usually meant that there were not enough physicians to round on hospital inpatients and furnish nonhospital services in the community.

In addition to modifying the levels of supervision required for hospital outpatient services, CMS also modified this requirement to give hospitals and physicians more breathing room. Effective in 2011, CMS allows the supervising physician or NPP to be located off the hospital campus, or "in or near hospital buildings that house multiple provider-based departments, provided that they are immediately available" (*Medicare Benefit Policy Manual*, Chapter 6 §20.5, 2014). Therefore, currently, there is no limitation on the location of the supervising physician per se. As long as the physician meets the other requirements listed above, including the mandate that the physician be immediately available, the supervising physician or NPP may be located in the actual department, on the hospital campus, or in nonhospital property close to the hospital. This includes any location in a building off campus that houses multiple provider-based departments.

Coverage of Hospital Outpatient Diagnostic Services

Hospitals frequently furnish diagnostic services to Medicare beneficiaries in provider-based departments, in addition to therapeutic services. For example, hospitals may operate clinical laboratories, radiology departments, and various other diagnostic centers (e.g., stress testing, neuro-diagnostics, sleep laboratories) in outpatient departments. CMS defines diagnostic services as:

> *"An examination or procedure to which the patient is subjected, or which is performed on materials derived from a hospital outpatient, to obtain information to aid in the assessment of a medical condition or the identification of a disease. Among these examinations and tests are diagnostic laboratory services such as hematology and chemistry, diagnostic x-rays, isotope studies, EKGs, pulmonary function studies, thyroid function tests, psychological tests, and other tests given to determine the nature and severity of an ailment or injury."*
>
> —*Medicare Benefit Policy Manual, Chapter 6 §20.4, 2011.*

Similar to therapeutic services, Medicare has specific coverage requirements for diagnostic services furnished in hospital outpatient departments (42 *CFR* §410.28, 2011). The general coverage rules are similar, but not identical, to the coverage rules discussed above for therapeutic services. As detailed below, the general coverage rule mandates that diagnostic services are furnished:

- Directly or under arrangements by the hospital

- Under the order of a physician or NPP

- Under the appropriate level of supervision

Some diagnostic services are not covered under the general diagnostic coverage requirements and have their own coverage requirements, including:

- Cardiovascular and diabetes disease screening tests (42 *CFR* §§410.17, 410.18, 2011)

- Ultrasound screening for abdominal aortic aneurysm (42 *CFR* §410.19, 2011)

- Bone mass measurement (42 *CFR* §410.31, 2011)

- Screening and diagnostic mammography (42 *CFR* §410.34, 2011)

- Colorectal cancer screening tests (42 *CFR* §410.37, 2011)

- Prostate cancer screening tests (42 *CFR* §410.39, 2011)

- Screening pelvic examinations (42 *CFR* §410.56, 2011)

We discuss some of the coverage rules for these diagnostic services below, as well as some nuances for other diagnostic tests. However, it is important for the hospital to carefully review the regulations for all diagnostic examinations to ensure that everyone involved is aware of the specific coverage requirements for these services, including any limitations on the frequency that these may be covered.

Note that we are again referring here to the facility component of the diagnostic services furnished to Medicare beneficiaries, which are furnished by the hospital (including provider-based departments). We are not including in this discussion the professional services furnished to the patient by physicians and other nonphysician practitioners who bill separately for these services. Payment for facility services is separate and distinct from payment for professional services. Therefore, do not make the mistake of confusing the facility component of diagnostic services with the professional component of these services when reviewing the Medicare coverage rules discussed below.

Hospitals must comply with three primary requirements to ensure that these services are covered by Medicare in hospital outpatient departments. These requirements are detailed below.

Furnished directly or under arrangements by the hospital

This requirement is nearly identical to the first criteria for coverage of therapeutic services. The only additional consideration is that for specific diagnostic services to be covered, they must be ordinarily furnished by the hospital to its outpatients for diagnostic study and would be covered as inpatient services if furnished to an inpatient (42 *CFR* §410.28[a][2], [3], 2011; *Medicare Benefit Policy Manual*, Chapter 6, §20.4.4, 2014). CMS broadly defines the coverage for diagnostic examinations at 42 *CFR* §409.16(c) (2011) and the *Medicare Benefit Policy Manual*, Chapter 1 §50 (2014). At this point, covered inpatient diagnostic services appear to include all Part B covered diagnostic services described in 42 *CFR* Part 410. However, hospitals should monitor and carefully review the coverage for each diagnostic examination to ensure that the test is covered on both an inpatient and outpatient basis before the examination is offered to patients.

Physician's order

As outlined below, the requirements for physician orders vary from one diagnostic service to another. Some of these rules are summarized below. However, it is very important that hospitals review the actual regulations and manual provisions governing each diagnostic service to ensure that the correct coverage rules are followed.

General rule

With limited exceptions, diagnostic services are covered by Medicare in hospital outpatient departments only if they are ordered by a physician or NPP with clinical privileges at the hospital (see, e.g., 42 *CFR* §410.28[f], 2011; 42 *CFR* §410.32[a], 2011; 42 *CFR* §482.12[c][1], 2011;

42 *CFR* §482.26[b][4], 2011; 42 *CFR* §482.53[d][4], 1999). This is true even for services where the state law allows the test to be performed by laboratories and other diagnostic centers when self-referred by the patient. For example, in many—if not all—states, laboratories are allowed to process fecal occult blood testing submitted by an individual without a physician's order. The laboratory must charge the patient, or possibly a private health insurer, for this service. However, the hospital may not bill Medicare for that service, since there is no physician's order for the service, and, therefore, the service is not covered by Medicare. If the service is billed to, and reimbursed by, Medicare, these payments could be considered overpayments to the hospital.

This rule also leads to the implication that diagnostic exams may not be ordered for hospital outpatients by community physicians who do not have hospital privileges. This conforms with the CMS requirements that the hospital have an organized medical staff that establishes bylaws that limit provision of services to physicians and NPPs that have hospital privileges (42 *CFR* §§482.12[a], [c][1], 2011; 42 *CFR* §482.22, 2011).

For the most part, Medicare will cover diagnostic tests ordered by NPPs. However, physicians must order diagnostic mammograms for Medicare to cover this service (42 *CFR* §410.34[b][1], 2011). Therefore, Medicare will not cover these services if they are ordered by NPPs.

Exceptions to general rule—stricter treating physician ordering rule

Coverage of certain diagnostic services, including clinical laboratory tests and bone mass measurement, is even more limited. Specifically, Medicare will only cover such services if they are ordered by the practitioner who is treating the patient and uses the results in the management of the patient's medical condition (42 *CFR* §§410.28[f], 2011; 42 *CFR* §410.32[a], 2011). This is the treating practitioner order rule.

If the service is ordered by a physician who is not the patient's treating physician or an NPP, then the service will not be covered by Medicare. When auditing this requirement, the key is ensuring that the same physician who ordered the test is also receiving the test results and using those results to manage the patient's medical condition. For example, the physician who orders a glucose level for a diabetic patient must also be the same physician who receives the result and adjusts the patient's insulin or diet in response to the test result. In general, if one physician orders the test and a different physician receives the results and acts on them, this would not be covered by Medicare.

Exceptions to general rule—more liberal rules

Medicare covers services without a physician order in extremely rare circumstances. Screening mammograms are covered even if a patient self-refers for the service (42 *CFR* §410.34[c], 2011; *Medicare Benefit Policy Manual,* Chapter 15 §280.3, 2014). Therefore, Medicare beneficiaries may present to a hospital outpatient mammography department without a physician's order and still receive a covered screening mammogram.

Appropriate supervision

Like therapeutic services, Medicare covers diagnostic services only if they are furnished under the correct level of supervision (*Medicare Benefit Policy Manual*, Chapter 6 §20.4.4, 2014). The level of supervision for each diagnostic service is defined in the MPFS. The levels of supervision are:

- General supervision, indicated by a "1" on the MPFS

- Direct supervision, indicated by a "2" on the MPFS

- Personal supervision, indicated by a "3" on the MPFS

  —*Medicare Benefit Policy Manual*, Chapter 15 §80, 2014.

The definitions for these levels of supervision are detailed above under the discussion about therapeutic services.

Unlike therapeutic services, only physicians may supervise hospital staff in the performance of diagnostic services. NPPs may not perform this supervision. However, NPPs may personally perform specified diagnostic services, if allowed under their state scope of practice (*Medicare Benefit Policy Manual*, Chapter 6 §§20.4.4, 2014; *Medicare Benefit Policy Manual*, Chapter 15 §80, 2014). In that case, the NPP is only required to have the level of supervision required by Medicare for coverage of that NPP's services. For example, nurse practitioners are required by Medicare to work in collaboration with a physician (42 *CFR* §410.75[c][3], 2011). The following are the diagnostic tests which may be furnished by NPPs under Medicare coverage rules:

- Diagnostic tests personally performed by a qualified audiologist (42 *CFR* §410.32[b][2][ii], 2011)

- Diagnostic psychological testing personally furnished by a clinical psychologist (42 *CFR* §410.32[b][2][iii], 2011)

- Diagnostic tests performed by specialty qualified physical therapists as permitted under state law (42 *CFR* §410.32[b][2][iv], 2011)

- Diagnostic tests performed by a nurse practitioner, clinical nurse specialist, a certified nurse midwife, or a physician's assistant as permitted under state law (42 *CFR* §410.32[b] [2][v], (vii), 2011; 42 *CFR* §410.32[b][3], 2011)

The only exceptions to the supervision rule are diagnostic mammography, which is regulated by the Food and Drug Administration (FDA), and laboratory and pathology services in the 80000 series of the current procedural terminology codes. These services are not required to be furnished under any specific level of supervision.

 © 2015 HCPro

Coverage of Outpatient Drugs

Coverage for drugs under Medicare Part B is fairly limited. However, Medicare does cover drugs that are administered "incident to" a physician's services and that:

- *"Meet the definition of drugs or biologicals (see §50.1)*
- *Are of the type that are not usually self-administered (see §50.2)*
- *Meet all the general requirements for coverage of items as "incident to" a physician's services (see §§50.1 and 50.3)*
- *Are reasonable and necessary for the diagnosis or treatment of the illness or injury for which they are administered according to accepted standards of medical practice (see §50.4)*
- *Are not excluded as non-covered immunizations (see §50.4.4.2)*
- *Have not been determined by the FDA to be less than effective. (See §50.4.4)."*

  —Medicare Benefit Policy Manual, Chapter 15 §§50, 2014.

Drugs that are "usually self-administered"

In general, Medicare does not cover drugs that are usually self-administered (self-administered drugs, or SAD) except in limited circumstances (*Medicare Benefit Policy Manual*, Chapter 15 §§50, 50.2, 50.5, 2014). The MAC is charged by CMS with making the determination as to whether a drug is "usually self-administered" (*Medicare Benefit Policy Manual*, Chapter 15 §§50.2, 2014). This determination is not made on a patient by patient basis and, instead, is made for each drug based on the following specific criteria:

- With some limited exceptions, drugs administered in any manner other than injection or infusion are considered to be usually self-administered and not covered (*Medicare Benefit Policy Manual*, Chapter 15 §§50.2[B], 2014). This includes drugs administered orally, by suppository, and topically.

- Drugs administered by subcutaneous injection are presumed to be usually self-administered (*Medicare Benefit Policy Manual*, Chapter 15 §§50.2[C]3, 2014). This includes, for example, insulin given to treat diabetes. However, this is a rebuttable presumption, and MACs may cover a drug that is administered subcutaneously if there is evidence that the drug is usually given for an acute condition and based on the frequency of administration.

- Drugs administered intravenously or by intramuscular injection are presumed to not be "usually self-administered" (*Medicare Benefit Policy Manual*, Chapter 15 §§50.2(C) 1 & 2, 2014).

The current SAD list is published on the CMS Coverage Center, which contains the drugs that the MACs have determined to be usually self-administered (*www.cms.gov/medicare-coverage-database/reports/sad-exclusion-list-report.aspx?bc=AQAAAAAAAAAAA%3d%3d&*). This database is called the "Self-Administered (SAD) Exclusion List Report" and allows the user to search for particular drugs under the local MAC.

Coverage of drugs that are "usually self-administered"

As noted above, CMS does not usually cover drugs that are usually self-administered. However, CMS does cover drugs that are usually self-administered in an outpatient hospital setting under the following conditions:

- **Statutorily-covered drugs.** Certain drugs are expressly covered under Medicare under specific statutory authority (*Medicare Benefit Policy Manual*, Chapter 15 §50.5, 2014). For example, Medicare coverage for the following drugs is authorized by Congress:

  - Drugs used in immunosuppressive therapy (*Medicare Benefit Policy Manual*, Chapter 15 §50.5.1, 2014)

  - Erythropoietin for dialysis patients (*Medicare Benefit Policy Manual*, Chapter 15 §50.5.2, 2014)

  - Certain oral anti-cancer drugs and anti-emetics used for specific medical conditions (*Medicare Benefit Policy Manual*, Chapter 15 §§50.5.3 & 50.5.4, 2014)

  - Hemophilia clotting factors (*Medicare Benefit Policy Manual*, Chapter 15 §50.5.4, 2014)

  The hospital should review the specific requirements for these drugs, since the coverage criteria are detailed in the statute and implementing regulations.

- **Drugs furnished integral to procedures.** Medicare covers certain self-administered drugs if they are administered to the patient as an integral part of a procedure or are directly related to the procedure (*Medicare Benefit Policy Manual*, Chapter 15 §50.5.2[M]). Put another way, Medicare covers a drug in the very few circumstances when the drug is treated as an essential supply for completion of the procedure (i.e., when the drug facilitates the performance of or recovery from a particular procedure) (*Medicare Benefit Policy Manual*, Chapter 15 §50.5.2[M], 2014). CMS gives the following examples of the types of drugs that may be covered under this criterion:

  - *"Sedatives administered to a patient while he or she is in the preoperative area being prepared for a procedure.*

  - *Mydriatic drops instilled into the eye to dilate the pupils, anti-inflammatory drops, antibiotic drops/ointments, and ocular hypotensives that are administered to a patient immediately before, during, or immediately following an ophthalmic procedure. This does not refer to the patient's eye drops that the patient uses pre and postoperatively.*

– *Barium or low osmolar contrast media provided integral to a diagnostic imaging procedure.*

– *Topical solution used with photodynamic therapy furnished at the hospital to treat non-hyperkeratotic actinic keratosis lesions of the face or scalp.*

– *Antibiotic ointments such as bacitracin, placed on a wound or surgical incision at the completion of a procedure."*

—*Medicare Benefit Policy Manual,* Chapter 15 §50.2[M], 2014.

Except for the applicable copayment, hospitals may not bill beneficiaries for these types of drugs, because their costs, as supplies, are packaged into the payment for the procedure with which they are used.

CMS has furnished another list of drugs that would not be considered integral to a procedure to assist hospitals in differentiating covered and non-covered drugs:

– *"Drugs given to a patient for his or her continued use at home after leaving the hospital.*

– *Oral pain medication given to an outpatient who develops a headache while receiving chemotherapy administration treatment.*

– *Daily routine insulin or hypertension medication given preoperatively to a patient.*

– *A fentanyl patch or oral pain medication such as hydrocodone, given to an outpatient presenting with pain.*

– *A laxative suppository for constipation while the patient waits to receive an unrelated x-ray."*

—*Medicare Benefit Policy Manual,* Chapter 15 §50.2M

As you can see from these lists, CMS intends to limit coverage of drugs under this exception and will treat the vast majority of drugs that are usually self-administered as non-covered.

Scenarios

The following scenarios may assist in better understanding the Medicare coverage requirements covered in this chapter.

Scenario A

You are performing an audit of the new preventive medicine provider-based clinic and are focusing on whether the services are furnished in accordance with the Medicare coverage requirements. The nursing staff tell you that the services are never supervised by a physician and that they furnish the following services in the clinic:

- Influenza, hepatitis B, and pneumococcal vaccination clinics

- Kidney disease education services

You are concerned that the lack of physician supervision for these services will cause a problem meeting the Medicare "incident to" coverage requirements.

Response:

Neither of the services listed are subject to the Medicare "incident to" coverage rule. Both of these services are therapeutic services. However, these services are exempt from the "incident to" coverage rules, because they are covered under separate coverage rules that do not require physician supervision.

Scenario B

When auditing the infusion clinic, the nursing staff tells you that the clinic is open 8 a.m.–10 p.m. every day of the week except Sunday. You ask for the schedule for the supervising physician and find that there is no supervising physician scheduled 8–10 p.m. daily or on Saturdays. However, there is a medical director for the clinic who furnishes general supervision for the clinic.

The clinic provides the following services:

- C8957 Prolonged IV infusion requiring pump

- 36430 Blood transfusion service

- 36591 Draw blood off venous device

- 96365 Ther/proph/diag IV infusion initial, up to one hour

You are concerned that the lack of physician supervision for these services at certain hours will cause a problem meeting the Medicare "incident to" coverage requirements for these therapeutic services.

Response:

When you research these services on the CMS list of "Hospital Outpatient Therapeutic Services That Have Been Evaluated for a Change in Supervision Level," you find that two of these services—36430 (blood transfusion service) and 36591 (draw blood off venous device)—require general physician supervision.

 © 2015 HCPro

Since the clinic is furnishing these services under a general level of supervision, this meets the supervision coverage requirement for these services.

You see that the other two services—96365 (ther/proph/diag IV infusion initial, up to one hour) and C8957 (prolonged IV infusion requiring pump)—require an NSEDTS level of supervision. This means that the services must be initiated under a direct level of supervision, then may be furnished under a general level of supervision if and when the supervising physician documents that the patient is stable and may be moved to that level of supervision. Given that the supervising physician is not available at all during certain hours, there is a risk that this level of supervision is not being met. Therefore, remediation is required in this clinic. Furthermore, there is a risk that these services have been furnished in the past for Medicare beneficiaries in violation of this requirement, and the hospital may need to consult with legal counsel to determine if there is an overpayment that must be disclosed and repaid.

Scenario C

When auditing the wound care clinic, you review two records, with the following findings:

- Patient A has an order for wound care for a right ankle ulcer three times a week for 10 weeks. The nurses documented that the wound had worsened in week three and decided to have the patient come in for an extra visit that week. During that same visit, the patient pointed out a new ulcer on her left big toe, so the nurse implemented the same wound care orders for the new ulcer. There are no physician visits or additional orders for the full 10 weeks. When the nurse is interviewed, she states that she has worked with the patient's treating physician for many years and knows that is what the physician would have ordered. The patient's ulcers heal well, and the patient was very satisfied with the care delivered.

- Patient B has orders written by Physician X for a lab test. The results of the lab test are ordered to be delivered to Physician Y, who reviews the results and implements the correct therapeutic drug for the condition.

You note that both patients are doing very well, but have some concerns about whether the Medicare coverage requirements are met for these services.

Response:

After researching the Medicare coverage requirements for therapeutic and diagnostic services, you arrive at the following conclusions:

- There is a risk that Patient A's wound care may not be covered by Medicare, because the services were not furnished in accordance with the "incident to" requirements. Specifically, the nurse failed to refer the patient back to the physician for a personal reassessment of the worsening ulcer and an assessment of the new ulcer, which meant that the services were not furnished as an "integral, although incidental" part of the physician's services. The nurse also failed to obtain a physician's order for the additional visits and the services furnished for new ulcer. This violates not only the physician order requirement under the "incident to" coverage requirements, but also the nurse's state scope of practice.

- There is a risk that Patient B's lab test may not be covered by Medicare because this clinical diagnostic lab test was not ordered by the "treating physician." The physician who ordered the test was not the same physician who received the results and treated the patient based on the results of the test.

 © 2015 HCPro

Billing and Reimbursement for Services Furnished in Provider-Based Departments

Overview

After studying the provider-based criteria in the prior chapters, you probably want to get started on auditing your current hospital operations for compliance. However, you are not ready to audit your hospital-based departments until you understand how to properly code and bill for these services. Comprehending and preparing to implement the new requirements for the -PO modifier and POS coding effective in 2016 are especially important in this regard.

In addition, hospitals should understand the difference between the reimbursement for services furnished in provider-based departments and freestanding facilities. This is useful to better perform cost-benefit analyses when acquiring freestanding facilities and to determine if the acquisition is financially advantageous given the additional costs of compliance involved with provider-based departments. This knowledge is also helpful in better comprehending CMS' concerns about provider-based departments and communicating that concern with some urgency to hospital and medical staff leadership when trying to enforce compliance in this area.

Finally, hospitals must not assume that the provision of services in a provider-based department has no impact on Medicare beneficiaries. In that regard, the hospital must be prepared to explain to Medicare beneficiaries how the use of provider-based departments may increase their cost-sharing liability. This is especially important if the hospital is incorporating a freestanding clinic that has been in operation for a period of time, because the patients of that facility will be continuing their care in the newly designated provider-based hospital department, and must be made aware of potential billing changes.

Overall, the coding and billing for provider-based departments is changing very little, with two exceptions. Beginning in 2016, hospitals must add the -PO modifier to all UB-04 Uniform Bill institutional claims for services furnished in off-campus provider-based departments. In addition, beginning in 2016, different POS codes will be required on CMS 1500 professional services claims to distinguish between services furnished in on-campus and off-campus provider-based clinics. CMS is implementing these changes to gather information about the type and volume of services furnished in off-campus provider-based departments. With this vast database of information, CMS will be able to more easily find billing errors, benchmark these services, and focus audits on hospitals that appear to perform a higher number of off-campus services.

Components of Services

In general, there are two ingredients or "components" of medical services: the professional component and the facility/technical component. The professional component refers to the hands-on services furnished by the physicians and NPPs. This includes evaluation and management (E/M) services such as the assessment of the patient, review of test results, education and counseling, and determination of the plan of care. Surgeries and other procedures personally performed by physicians and NPPs are also included in this component.

The facility or technical component encompasses everything that contributes to the medical care aside from the professional services. This includes payment for staff who furnish hands-on nursing care, infusions, medication administration, education, counseling, and other nonphysician services, such as the technical portion of diagnostic and therapeutic services. This component also includes the overhead costs necessary to operate the clinic and furnish the services, such as the costs of the supplies, medication, building, utilities, administrative staff, laundry, security, medical records, and contracted services.

Components of services furnished in freestanding physician offices

When a service is performed in a freestanding physician office, the physician or medical group generally furnishes and incurs the costs of the entire service, including both the professional and facility/technical components. The physician operating the freestanding office is responsible for the facility/technical costs of furnishing each service, including but not limited to payment for the following:

- Utilities, maintenance, and other facility expenses for the office building

- Lease or mortgage expenses

- Taxes

- Clerical and billing staff salaries and benefits

 © 2015 HCPro

- Nursing staff salaries and benefits

- Medical supplies

- Drugs

- Medical equipment

- Diagnostic machines

When the patient receives services in a freestanding physician office, he or she generally uses both facility/technical services (e.g., the treatment room, supplies, equipment) and professional services (i.e., services provided directly by the NPP and physician). However, there are occasions when the patient receives services that do not involve the physician's professional services, such as when the nurse personally performs a dressing change or an in-office lab test without the need for physician involvement. In those cases, there is no professional component of the service furnished to the patient, because the service did not require any effort by the physician. However, in any case, the physician or medical group incurs the cost of the facility/technical component of these services, including the nursing staff, equipment, and building.

Because the physician or medical group incurs the costs for both the facility and professional services when a patient is seen in a freestanding office, the physician or medical group is entitled to bill Medicare globally for both components of the service. Generally, there is only one line item for each billable service on the claim, and this line item claim constitutes the charge for the entire service. In addition, there is generally only one claim for the services; no separate claim should be submitted by any hospital or other facility for these services. This is true for all types of services—therapeutic and diagnostic.

Freestanding offices are subject to fewer state and federal regulations. Therefore, they do not have to incur the cost of audits and surveys or the increased cost of the complex compliance schemes required for provider-based entities. Freestanding facilities are not usually required to be accredited, and typically do not have to comply with complex building and earthquake code requirements. Therefore, the facility costs for these entities are usually much lower than in provider-based departments.

Components of services furnished in a provider-based department

Unlike a freestanding physician office, the professional and facility components of medical services are split-billed for provider-based departments, because these components are furnished by two separate entities: the hospital and the physician/medical group. Even though the services furnished by both the hospital and the physician/medical group in provider-based department are covered under Medicare Part B, each entity must bill the services separately on different types of claim forms. There are limited exceptions to this split-billing methodology. Under certain CMS pilot projects, the hospital bills for both components and then is responsible for sharing the reimbursement with the physicians. In addition, CAHs may choose alternative billing methodologies that allow them to bill for both components and reimburse the physicians directly. These exceptions are not discussed further here.

When services are furnished in a provider-based department, the facility/technical component of the service is furnished by the hospital. This is because the hospital contributes to the provision of services by employing the nursing and clerical staff, owning or leasing the building where the services are provided, purchasing the medical supplies and equipment, and maintaining the medical record. Therefore, unlike in the freestanding physician office, there are separate charges for the facility component of the services at the provider-based department, and the hospital is entitled to bill separately for these facility services. The hospital should bill Medicare for these services on a UB-04 claim form (837I electronic billing form) under its own name and billing identifiers.

The physicians and NPPs who furnish the professional component of the medical services are entitled to separately bill Medicare for the professional services under their name and Medicare billing number on the CMS-1500 claim form (837P electronic billing form). This is identical to the billing that would be required if the services had been performed in the freestanding physician office. However, since the hospital furnishes the facility/technical component of the services, the physician may not bill for that component of the services, and only the hospital is entitled to do so. Instead, the physician is limited to billing for the professional component, which reflects the personal work effort expended by the physician to perform the services.

Some services furnished in a provider-based department have a facility component but not a professional component. These are services that are performed solely by the hospital personnel and do not involve any personal services by the physician or NPP. For example, after an initial physician evaluation, a course of wound care or infusions ordered by the physician may be performed over a period of time by the nursing staff with physician oversight and supervision even if the physician does not perform any personal services. In this instance, the provider-based department may only bill the facility component, since there was no professional service furnished by the physician. The hospital alone may bill for these services, just like the other facility services it furnished.

As noted previously, the costs of furnishing facility/technical services in a provider-based department are naturally much higher than the costs of those same services provided in a freestanding physician office. Hospitals are highly regulated by state and federal governments, which means that they are subject to multiple complex regulations, including, for example, requirements to maintain an organized medical staff and specific documentation in the medical record, as well as to comply with life safety and earthquake codes and EMTALA. Therefore, the overhead costs for services furnished in these types of providers are higher than similar services furnished in freestanding physician offices and other facilities.

Example of Differences in Billing Components: Freestanding Physician Office Versus Provider-Based Department

The following examples demonstrate the difference in billing for the same services furnished in a freestanding physician office (global billing) and a provider-based hospital outpatient department (split billing).

Service performed in a freestanding physician office

Consider a service performed in a freestanding physician office. Patient A has a visit at an orthopedic surgeon's freestanding office and is examined by the physician. A medical assistant performs an x-ray of the patient's affected leg and also performs an electrocardiogram (EKG). A registered nurse dresses the wound. A phlebotomist then draws the patient's blood in the phlebotomy station attached to the physician office in preparation for an upcoming surgery. The physician reviews and interprets the leg x-ray and the EKG, and documents the entire visit in the patient's physician office medical record. The laboratory specimen is sent to the laboratory at Hospital X across the street. This may result in the billing scenario outlined in Figure 6.1.

Figure 6.1	Billing Scenario for Services Performed in Freestanding Surgeon's Office					
Service	Surgeon Bills for Service			Hospital X Bills for Service		
	Technical/ Facility Component	Professional Component	Global	Technical/ Facility Component	Professional Component	Global
Physician Encounter (E/M Visit)			X			
X-Ray of Leg			X			
EKG			X			
Wound Dressing	X					
Blood Draw	X					
Laboratory Test						X

*Source: **Gina M. Reese, Esq., RN,** an instructor for HCPro's Medicare Boot Camp®—Hospital Version and Medicare Boot Camp®—Utilization Review Version. Reprinted with permission.*

In this case, the surgeon is able to bill for all the services except the actual performance of the laboratory test, because that was done in the laboratory located in Hospital X. The breakdown of billable services is as follows:

- The surgeon performed the E/M visit with the patient in his own facility, incurring both the professional cost of the service (his own time and work effort) as well as the facility component (the overhead of the building, equipment, staff assistance, and supplies). Therefore, he is able to bill this service globally on his claim.

- The x-ray and EKG were performed in the physician's office, and the surgeon himself interpreted these diagnostic tests, incurring the professional cost of the service (his personal work effort in interpreting the exams) as well as the facility component (the overhead of the building, equipment, staff assistance, and supplies). Therefore, the surgeon is also able to bill globally for these services.

- Note that there was no professional component for the wound dressing and the blood draw, since the service was furnished by the physician office staff with no hands-on participation by the surgeon. The surgeon still bills for these services, but they are reimbursed on a basis that reflects that they do not include a physician work effort.

- Hospital X may not bill for any of these services except the laboratory test, because it did not furnish these services or incur the cost of performing the services. Hospital X is able to bill for the laboratory test performed in its own laboratory, because it owns the laboratory and incurred the costs for performing that service.

Service performed in provider-based department

Contrast the discussion above with the situation where Patient B receives exactly the same services, but they are performed in a provider-based surgery outpatient department at Hospital X instead of a freestanding physician office. Again, the laboratory test is drawn in the department, but sent to Hospital X's laboratory, which obtains the results. The orthopedic surgeon is on the medical staff at Hospital X. He performs the E/M visit with the patient in that provider-based department and interprets the EKG and leg x-ray. The services are documented in the hospital medical record and may result in the billing scenario outlined in Figure 6.2.

 © 2015 HCPro

Figure 6.2	Billing Scenario for Services Performed in Provider-Based Department at Hospital X					
Service	Surgeon Bills for Service			Hospital X Bills for Service		
	Technical/Facility Component	Professional Component	Global	Technical/Facility Component	Professional Component	Global
Physician Encounter (E/M Visit)		X		X		
X-Ray of Leg		X		X		
EKG		X		X		
Wound Dressing				X		
Blood Draw				X		
Laboratory Test						X

Source: *Gina M. Reese, Esq., RN,* an instructor for HCPro's Medicare Boot Camp®—Hospital Version and Medicare Boot Camp®—Utilization Review Version. Reprinted with permission.

This example demonstrates split billing for some of these services, which means the hospital bills for the facility/technical component of therapeutic and diagnostic services, and the surgeon bills for the professional component of those services. In this scenario, Hospital X bills for all services except the professional component of the physician E/M visit, as well as the professional components of the x-ray and EKG, which were interpreted by the physician. The breakdown of billable services is as follows:

- The surgeon bills for the professional component of the E/M visit and the interpretations of the diagnostic tests.

- Hospital X bills for the facility component of the E/M visit as well as the diagnostic x-ray and EKG, because the hospital furnished and incurred the cost for the building, equipment, and staff that performed the nonprofessional portion of those services.

- Note that there was no professional component for the wound dressing and the blood draw, since these services were furnished by the hospital clinical staff with no hands-on participation by the surgeon. Therefore, Hospital X will bill for the facility/technical services associated with these services.

- Just like in the scenario above, the hospital bills for the laboratory test performed in its own laboratory, because it owns the laboratory and incurred the costs for performing that service.

E/M service performed in freestanding physician office and diagnostic and other services furnished in provider-based department

Another variation of this scenario could involve a patient who is seen by the physician in a freestanding physician office for the E/M visit. In this instance, the physician sends the patient to Hospital X for the diagnostic testing and wound care, and the diagnostic tests are interpreted by hospital-based physicians on the medical staff. This may result in the billing scenario outlined in Figure 6.3.

Figure 6.3	Billing Scenario When E/M Performed in Freestanding Physician Office; Other Services Performed in Provider-Based Department at Hospital X								
Service	Surgeon Bills for Service			Hospital X Bills for Service			Interpreting Physician Bills		
	Technical/ Facility Compo-nent	Profes-sional Com-ponent	Global	Technical/ Facility Compo-nent	Profes-sional Com-ponent	Global	Technical/ Facility Compo-nent	Profes-sional Com-ponent	Global
Physician Encounter (E/M Visit)		X							
X-Ray of Leg				X				X	
EKG				X				X	
Wound Dressing				X					
Blood Draw				X					
Laboratory Test						X			

*Source: **Gina M. Reese, Esq., RN**, an instructor for HCPro's Medicare Boot Camp®—Hospital Version and Medicare Boot Camp®—Utilization Review Version. Reprinted with permission.*

This example demonstrates another type of split billing whereby the hospital bills for the facility/technical component of the diagnostic services, and the interpreting physicians bill for the professional component of those services. In this scenario, Hospital X again ends up billing for all of the services except the professional component of the physician E/M visit and the professional components of the x-ray and EKG, which were interpreted by the physician. The breakdown of billable services is as follows:

- The surgeon only bills for the professional component of the E/M visit since that was the only service furnished by the surgeon.

- Hospital X bills for the facility component of the diagnostic x-ray and EKG, since the hospital furnished and incurred the cost for the building, equipment, and staff that performed the nonprofessional portion of those services.

- Note that there was no professional component for the wound dressing and the blood draw, since the service was furnished by the hospital clinical staff with no hands-on participation by the surgeon. Therefore, these are billed just by Hospital X.

- The hospital-based physicians on the medical staff who interpreted the EKG and leg x-ray bill for the professional component of these services, because they furnished the personal work effort for these services. They would bill for these services on a CMS 1500 form under their own names and billing numbers.

- Just like in the scenarios above, the hospital still bills for the laboratory test performed in its own laboratory, because it owns the laboratory and incurred the costs for performing that service.

Notably, in this scenario, there would be three or more claims submitted for these services, rather than just the two claims submitted in the two prior scenarios. In the prior scenarios, there would be one claim submitted by the surgeon and one claim submitted by Hospital X.

However, the following occurs with regard to the third scenario:

- The surgeon submits a claim for the professional component of the E/M visit

- Hospital X submits a claim for the technical component of the services furnished at the hospital as well as the lab test

- At a minimum, two interpreting physicians submit claims for the professional component of the interpreted exams

Reimbursement for Services in Freestanding Physician Offices

Services furnished by physicians and NPPs in freestanding physician offices and billed on the CMS 1500 claim form are reimbursed to the physicians/NPPs based on the MPFS (42 *USC* 1395w–4, n.d.; 42 *CFR* §414.1 et seq., 2015; *Medicare Claims Processing Manual*, Chapter 12, 2014). As discussed above, the professional claim for services is a global bill for the entire service—both the facility and professional component (if any) of each service are considered to be included on one line item on the claim. As detailed by a 2015 OIG audit report, the physician receives the "non-facility practice expense" fee schedule amount for the service:

> *"Medicare pays for physician services under the Social Security Act (the Act). The act requires that the fee schedule base the payments on national uniform relative value units (RVUs) according to the categories of costs used in furnishing a service.*

> *Medicare payment for physician services is based on the lower of the actual charge or the fee schedule amount. CMS publishes yearly updates to the fee schedule in the Federal Register …*

> *Federal requirements state: 'The non-facility PE [practice expense] RVUs apply to services performed in a physician's office, a patient's home, a nursing facility, or a facility or institution other than a hospital or skilled nursing facility, community mental health center, or ASC (42 CFR §414.22[b][5][i][B]).'*

—Incorrect Place-of-Service Claims, 2015.

The end result is that the reimbursement for a service furnished in a freestanding physician office (or, for that matter, in a patient's home or other place of residence) is paid to the physician at a higher rate than if he performs the same service in a hospital. As the OIG discussed in a 2015 report, this makes sense, because when a physician furnishes the services in his or her own office, he or she incurs the cost of the facility/technical component of the services, and therefore deserves the higher reimbursement for those services:

> *"Practice expense includes the overhead costs involved in providing a service. To account for the increased practice expense that physicians generally incur by performing services in their offices and other non-facility locations, Medicare reimburses physicians at a higher rate for certain services performed in these locations."*

—Incorrect Place-of-Service Claims, 2015.

Notably, as demonstrated in the tables above, when services are furnished in a freestanding physician office and no portion of these services are performed by the hospital, the hospital does not bill or receive reimbursement for any portion of the service in this location. This is true even if the hospital owns this location as a freestanding entity.

Reimbursement for Facility and Professional Services in a Provider-Based Department

As discussed above, services furnished in a provider-based department are generally billed in two or more claims—so-called split billing. A portion of the payment is made for the claim submitted by the hospital for its facility services, and the remainder is made for the claim for professional services provided by the physician or NPP. Of course, as noted above, there are certain services for which there is no professional component. In those cases, the hospital receives all of the reimbursement for these facility services.

There has historically been a fundamental difference between the amount of reimbursement paid by Medicare for services furnished in a freestanding physician office and the same services furnished in a provider-based department. CMS explained this in the recent regulation requiring the use of the new -PO modifier and POS codes:

> *"When a Medicare beneficiary receives outpatient services in a hospital, the total*
> *payment amount for outpatient services made by Medicare is generally higher than*
> *the total payment amount made by Medicare when a physician furnishes those*
> *same services in a freestanding clinic or in a physician office."*
>
> —*79 Fed. Reg. 66770, 66910, 2014.*

This increased reimbursement is due to the increased facility component paid to the hospital.

Professional component

The professional components of services furnished in the provider-based departments and billed on the CMS 1500 form are generally submitted by and paid separately to the physician or medical group based on the MPFS. This payment is based on the MPFS, just like the payment made for services in a freestanding physician office. However, the physicians who provide these services are supposed to be paid using the "facility practice expense" revenue value unit (RVU) methodology in the MPFS.

> *"The facility PE [practice expense] RVUs apply to services 'furnished to patients*
> *in the hospital, skilled nursing facility, community mental health center, or in an*
> *ambulatory surgical center.' (42 CFR §414.22[b][5][i][A])."*
>
> —Incorrect Place-of-Service Claims, 2015.

If paid correctly using this methodology, the physician receives a reduced portion of the MPFS amount to account for the fact that the services were furnished in the hospital outpatient department, rather than in the physician's office setting. The payment is reduced because the physician is not incurring the facility costs to furnish the service (*Medicare Claims Processing Manual*, Chapter 12, §20.4.2, 2014). Instead, these costs are being absorbed by the hospital, and the physician is only being reimbursed for the costs of his own professional services.

> *"For 2010 through 2012, nearly all physician services with payments that varied*
> *depending on place of service resulted in a higher payment when they were billed*
> *with a nonfacility place-of-service code."*
>
> —Incorrect Place-of-Service Claims, 2015.

Facility component

The services furnished by hospitals in provider-based departments are reimbursed under the Medicare payment scheme applicable to the main provider. For example, services furnished in a hospital outpatient department are paid under the hospital OPPS (42 *CFR* 419.1 et seq., 2015). In contrast, services provided to Medicare beneficiaries in CAHs are reimbursed at 101% of their reasonable costs (*Medicare Claims Processing Manual*, Chapter 3, §30.1.1, 2014).

When billing for services furnished in a provider-based department, the hospital is generally paid only for the facility or technical component of the services, which is billed to the MAC on the UB-04 claim form. The facility component is intended to reimburse the hospital for the services of the hospital staff as well as the supplies and overhead necessary to operate the clinic and furnish the services. The overhead costs for services furnished in provider-based departments are higher than similar services furnished in freestanding physician offices and other facilities. Therefore, the reimbursement for the facility component of these services is higher than if the services were furnished in a freestanding physician office.

Total reimbursement impact

The combined professional and facility payment for the services furnished in a provider-based department are generally more than the amount for the same services provided in a freestanding physician office. Even though the cost of the professional component is always lower in a provider-based entity, the hospital usually receives a larger facility payment under the OPPS that more than makes up for the decrease in the professional payment. In other words, as explained by CMS, this increased overall payment is attributable to an increased payment to the hospital and is designed to compensate the hospital for the higher overhead costs required to operate the provider-based clinic, which is more highly regulated than the freestanding physician clinic locations:

> "The total payment (including both Medicare program payment and beneficiary cost-sharing) generally is higher when outpatient services are furnished in the hospital outpatient setting rather than a freestanding clinic or a physician office. Both the OPPS and the MPFS establish payment based on the relative resources involved in furnishing a service. In general, we expect hospitals to have overall higher resource requirements than physician offices because hospitals are required to meet the conditions of participation, to maintain standby capacity for emergency situations, and to be available to address a wide variety of complex medical needs in a community. When services are furnished in the hospital setting such as in off-campus provider-based departments, Medicare pays the physician a lower facility payment under the MPFS, but then also pays the hospital under the OPPS. The beneficiary pays coinsurance for both the physician payment and the hospital outpatient payment. The term 'facility fee' refers to this additional hospital outpatient payment."

> —78 Fed. Reg. 43534, 43627, 2013.

Figures 6.4 and 6.5 illustrate two examples of this payment differential. In each example, we assume that the beneficiary has already met his or her annual deductible.

 © 2015 HCPro

Figure 6.4 outlines the difference in payment between a freestanding physician office and a provider-based department for a patient who is seen for simple clinic visit (CPT code 99213 for professional billing, G0463 for hospital outpatient billing) with a vaccination (CPT code 90471).

Figure 6.4	Differential Reimbursement for Simple Clinic Visit: Freestanding Physician Office Versus Provider-Based Clinic

Table A
Services Furnished in Freestanding Physician Office

Professional 837P Claim (POS =11)

Codes	MPFS Payment	Patient Copayment	Total Payment
99213	$56.90	$14.22	$71.12
90471	$19.73	$4.93	$24.66
Total Reimbursement	$76.63	$19.15	$95.78

Table B
Services Furnished in Provider-Based Department

Hospital 837I Claim			Professional 837P Claim (POS =22/19)			Total of Hospital and Professional Reimbursement
Codes	OPPS Payment	Patient Copayment	Codes	MPFS Payment	Patient Copayment	
G0463	$77.00	$19.25	99213	$40.02	$10.01	$146.28
90471	$42.83	$10.71	N/A	N/A	N/A	$53.54
Total Reimbursement	$119.83	$29.96		$40.02	$10.01	$199.82

Table C
Difference in Total Reimbursement
Services Furnished in Provider-Based Department versus Freestanding Physician Office

Total Payment in Provider-Based Department (Hospital + Professional)	Total Payment in Freestanding Physician Office (Professional Only)	Difference in Total Reimbursement
$199.82	$95.78	$104.04

Table D
Difference in Patient's Copayment
Services Furnished in Provider-Based Department versus Freestanding Physician Office

Copayment Provider-Based Clinic (Hospital + Professional)	Copayment Freestanding Physician Office (Professional Only)	Difference
$39.97	$19.15	$20.82

Source: *Gina M. Reese, Esq., RN, an instructor for HCPro's Medicare Boot Camp®—Hospital Version and Medicare Boot Camp®—Utilization Review Version. Reprinted with permission.*

In this example, the total payment to the physician is reduced by $45.75 in the provider-based setting, because the physician is not incurring any of the facility costs associated with the service. This payment differential is obtained by subtracting the total amount paid to the physician in a free-standing setting in Table A of Figure 6.4 ($76.63 in MPFS payment + $19.15 inpatient copayment = $95.78) and the total amount paid to the physician in the provider-based setting in Table B in Figure 6.4 ($40.02 in MPFS payment + $10.01 patient copayment = $50.03). This results in the following calculation: $95.78 - $50.03 = $45.75.

However, the hospital is paid $149.79 for this service under OPPS, which means that there is an additional $104.04 in reimbursement overall for this service (Medicare payments plus patient copayments) in this provider-based clinic as compared to the freestanding physician office.

This payment difference is significant enough for a simple clinic visit. However, Figure 6.5 illustrates a more complex example of this payment differential. In this instance, a patient is seen for a clinic visit (99213 for professional billing, G0463 for hospital outpatient billing) with a separately identifiable surgical procedure (excision of a lesion, CPT code 11420), which results in a higher differential.

Figure 6.5	Differential Reimbursement for Complex Clinic Visit: Freestanding Physician Office Versus Provider-Based Clinic

Table A
Services Furnished in Freestanding Physician Office

Professional 837P Claim (POS =11)			
Codes	MPFS Payment	Patient Copayment	Total Payment
99213-25	$56.90	$14.22	$71.12
11420	$129.18	$32.30	$161.48
Total Reimbursement	$186.08	$46.52	$232.60

Table B
Services Furnished in Provider-Based Department

Hospital 837I Claim			Professional 837P Claim (POS =22/19)			Total of Hospital and Professional Reimbursement
Codes	OPPS Payment	Patient Copayment	Codes	MPFS Payment	Patient Copayment	
G0463-25	$77.00	$19.25	99213-25	$40.02	$10.01	$146.28
11420	$302.84	$75.72	11420	$89.91	$22.48	$490.95
Total Reimbursement	$379.84	$94.97		$129.93	$32.48	$637.22

Table C
Difference in Total Reimbursement
Services Furnished in Provider-Based Department versus Free-Standing Physician Office

Total Payment in Provider-Based Department (Hospital + Professional)	Total Payment in Freestanding Physician Office (Professional Only)	Difference in Total Reimbursement
$637.22	$232.60	$404.62

Table D
Difference in Patient's Copayment
Services Furnished in Provider-Based Department vs. Freestanding Physician Office

Copayment Provider-Based Clinic (Hospital + Professional)	Copayment Freestanding Physician Office (Professional Only)	Difference
$127.45	$46.52	$106.63

Source: **Gina M. Reese, Esq., RN,** *an instructor for HCPro's* Medicare Boot Camp®–Hospital Version *and* Medicare Boot Camp®–Utilization Review Version. *Reprinted with permission.*

As you may see from Figure 6.5, the difference between the total reimbursement by Medicare for these particular services in the freestanding physician office ($232.60) and the provider-based facility ($637.22) is $404.63. It is easy to see that this payment differential could be more of an incentive for physicians and hospitals to collaborate and integrate their practices in order to obtain this higher overall rate of payment.

This payment differential is the source of most of the OIG and CMS concern about provider-based payments, and the resultant increased regulatory scrutiny of provider-based entities:

> *"Because the result can be an increase in costs supported by Medicare, 'with no commensurate benefit to Medicare and its beneficiaries,' CMS made clear that 'it is critical that CMS designate only those entities that are unquestionably qualified as provider-based.' "*

> —In the Case of Mira Vista, 2007.

CMS has expressed this concern in every regulation dealing with provider-based status (see, e.g., 63 *Fed. Reg.* 47552, 47588, 1998).

Interestingly, this payment differential may be reversing in favor of increased payment for services furnished in freestanding physician settings under the more recent OPPS payment methodology, effective in 2015, which increasingly packages payment for related ancillary services into the payment for the main clinic visit (*Medicare Claims Processing Manual*, Chapter 4 §10.4, 2015). This will not likely affect the payment differential that favors hospitals for simple clinic visits with few ancillary services. However, the more ancillary diagnostic and therapeutic services that are furnished, the more the balance tips in favor of higher payment in the freestanding physician office setting. This is because hospitals will no longer receive separate payments for the majority of related ancillary services furnished in the provider-based hospital departments. In comparison, physicians will still receive a separate payment for each of the services. The end result is that the freestanding physician office will receive a higher payment for these services. This is illustrated in a recent analysis in HCPro's *Medicare Insider* (see Figure 6.6).

© 2015 HCPro

Figure 6.6	Projected Reimbursement Under OPPS Payment Methodology Packaging More Ancillary Services

During a visit, a physician orders a chest x-ray (71010), complete blood count (85025), and spirometry (94010) for suspected pneumonia. That afternoon, the patient goes to the hospital radiology department for the chest x-ray, the laboratory for the CBC, and the pulmonology department for the spirometry.

Service	Freestanding (POS 11)	Provider-Based (POS 22/19)	Difference as PBD
Allowable for professional services (99214)	$108.34	$79.02	-$29.32
Allowable for facility services (G0463)	None	$96.25	$96.25
Allowable for the spirometry	$161.22	$0	-$161.22
Allowable for the chest x-ray	$0	$0	$0
Allowable for CBC	$0	$0	$0
Total Allowable	$269.56	$175.27	-$94.29

Note: The chest x-ray and CBC do not change the payment in the example, but are added to highlight the additional costs that may need to be borne by the hospital as additional testing is ordered.

The expanded example now shows a loss of $94 for the provider-based location, assuming the same services are provided in the same way, and the only difference is the manner in which the clinic location is treated for billing purposes: provider-based or freestanding. The reason for this difference is the increased packaging of ancillary services implemented in the OPPS for CY 2015. With these new rules, the finances of provider-based locations flip-flopped from an apparent profit to a loss, not even including the increased costs of operating as provider-based, discussed above.

Source: Adapted from Baker, K., Note from the Instructor: Provider-Based vs. Freestanding Locations: Financials Flip-Flop With New Packaging, Medicare Insider (May 12, 2015), www.hcpro.com/CCP-316291-5091/Note-from-the-Instructor-ProviderBased-vs-Freestanding-Locations-Financials-Flipflop-with-New-Packaging.html.

This change in reimbursement methodology may eventually take the pressure off of provider-based departments. However, until that occurs, providers must still ensure compliance with the provider-based requirements and the coding requirements.

More About Coding and Billing for Provider-Based Services

Professional component

As demonstrated in the tables above, when services are furnished in a provider-based department, the services are split billed; the physician or NPP bills for the professional component of services (if any), and the hospital bills for the facility or technical component. The professional component of the services furnished in provider-based departments is coded on the CMS 1500 claim form with the E/M or other CPT codes that best describe the services. For example, the range of CPT codes 99201–99205, 99211–99215, etc., would be applicable for coding of E/M services, and diagnostic services are billed using the 80000 series.

All applicable CPT coding rules apply when coding provider-based services, including the difference in coding for new and established patients. In addition, modifiers must be used as appropriate (*Medicare Claims Processing Manual*, Chapter 12, §30 et seq., 2014). For example, procedures and E/M services performed during the same encounter require modifier -25 on the E/M claim line item in situations when the E/M services are significant and separately identifiable from the procedure. As another example, the professional code for diagnostic tests with the exception of clinical laboratory tests require modifier -26.

Claims for the professional component of services must be coded in Field 24B on the CMS 1500 claim form with a POS code that describes the location where the services were furnished (*Medicare Claims Processing Manual*, Chapter 26 §10.5, 201, 2014; *Medicare Claims Processing Manual*, Chapter 12, §20.4.2, 2014). For example, professional services performed in an inpatient hospital setting are coded with POS code 21, whereas services furnished in a hospital outpatient department are coded with POS code 22, and those furnished in a freestanding physician office are coded with POS code 11. (More information on existing POS codes is available on the CMS website at: *www.cms.gov/Medicare/Coding/place-of-service-codes/Place_of_Service_Code_Set.html*.)

The MAC uses these POS codes for the following purposes:

- Matching the POS code with the hospital facility billing for that service. For example, if the POS code is 11, the MAC would not expect to receive a hospital facility claim for that service. In contrast, if the POS code is 21 or 22, the MAC would expect that the hospital would bill a facility component for that service (although there is not always a facility component).

- To determine the appropriate level of reimbursement for the professional services.

As noted by the OIG:

> *"Physicians are required to identify the place of service correctly on the claim forms that they submit to the Medicare contractors. The correct place-of-service code ensures that Medicare correctly reimburses the physician for the overhead portion of the service. Claim form instructions state that each physician is responsible for becoming familiar with Medicare coverage and billing requirements."*

> —Incorrect Place-of-Service Claims, 2015.

Historically, the oversight of the correct use of POS coding has not been rigorous. Therefore, the OIG has repeatedly reviewed the accuracy of POS coding and the resultant reimbursement for these services. Prior to its 2015 audit, the OIG conducted four nationwide audits of POS coding from 2009 through 2011, which resulted identifying nearly $63 million in overpayments to physicians due to misuse of POS coding (Incorrect Place-of-Service Claims, 2015). The OIG conducted 12 additional specific provider and contractor overpayment audits from 2003 and 2013, resulting in an additional approximately $73.5 million in overpayments.

For example, the OIG found in a review of the POS codes submitted to one MAC that:

> "Seventy-six of 100 sampled physician services, selected from a population of services identified as having a high potential for error, were performed in a facility but were billed by the physician using the 'office' or other non-facility place of service codes. As a result of the incorrect coding, Medicare paid the physicians a higher amount for these services. Based on a statistical projection, we estimate that [the MAC] overpaid physicians $1,051,477 for incorrectly coded services provided during a 2-year period ended December 31, 2002."
>
> —Review of Place of Service Coding for Physician Services, 2005.

The OIG originally attributed the overpayments to weak controls in Medicare payment systems. At that time, the Part B professional claim processing was performed in a separate system from the Part B outpatient hospital claim billing because two separate contractors processed these claims. Therefore, there was no systematic method of cross-checking the claims against each other for accuracy. Since that time, in accordance with the Medicare Prescription Drug, Improvement, and Modernization Act of 2003 (Public Law 108-173), the processing of these types of claims has been consolidated into one MAC, in part to establish better controls over these types of billing errors (Incorrect Place-of-Service Claims, 2015).

Although CMS is now able to better match professional bills with hospital outpatient bills using the POS codes, there continues to be misuse of the POS, causing continued overpayments. In a May 2015 audit, the OIG found continued abuse in this area, resulting in $33.4 million in overpayments for incorrectly coded services furnished between January 2010 and September 2012 (Incorrect Place-of-Service Claims, 2015).

Based on the continued failure of physicians to code the POS correctly, CMS decided to take additional steps to monitor the services furnished in off-campus provider-based departments, which are the most likely to be a source of abuse. The use of one POS code 22 for all hospital outpatient departments has not been effective in assisting CMS in determining the volume and types of services that are provided in each of these types of hospital outpatient departments. Therefore, CMS has been searching for tools to gather information about these services.

> *"In order to better understand the growing trend toward hospital acquisition of physician offices and subsequent treatment of those locations as off-campus provider-based outpatient departments, we are considering collecting information that would allow us to analyze the frequency, type, and payment for services furnished in off-campus provider-based hospital departments."*
>
> —*78 Fed. Reg. 43534, 43627, 2013.*

Therefore, CMS plans to require different POS codes to better distinguish between professional services furnished in on-campus and off-campus hospital settings (79 *Fed. Reg.* 66770, 66914, 2014). Effective January 1, 2016, POS 19 must be used on professional claims submitted for services furnished in off-campus departments, and POS 22 must be used solely for services furnished in on-campus hospital outpatient departments. (*Transmittal 3315,* Section I.B, August 6, 2015).

In combination with the -PO modifier, which will be required for provider-based billing, these new POS codes will allow CMS to gather more accurate and complete information about the volume and types of professional services furnished in provider-based settings. Of course, that means that CMS will be better armed to flag off-campus services for auditing and may eventually lead to a decrease in reimbursement for these services (79 *Fed. Reg.* 66770, 66910, 2014).

Facility component: coding for hospital-based services

The facility component of the hospital-based services is billed on the UB-04 billing form (837I electronic form) (42 *CFR* §424.32[b], 2012). Generally, one UB form is submitted for all related services provided on the same date during the same encounter. If multiple encounters occur on the same date (i.e., patient leaves premises and returns to same or different department), separate claims may be reported as long as all related services, including hospital services ordered by the physician as a result of the encounter, are combined on a single claim.

The facility component of hospital-based services is coded using:

- The HCPCS G-codes created by CMS (e.g., G0463 for clinic services)
- The same E/M and/or CPT codes used for professional billing
- Certain HCPCS Level II codes

More specifically, the facility component is coded as follows in this setting:

- Hospital outpatient clinic encounters are billed with HCPCS code G0463 (*Medicare Claims Processing Manual, Transmittal 2845,* 2013).
- Type A hospital emergency department (ED) visits, as defined by EMTALA, are billed using CPT Emergency Department Visit Codes (99281–99285). A Type A ED is a "dedicated emergency department" that is open 24 hours a day, 7 days a week. For this

purpose, a dedicated ED is a facility that is licensed by the state as an ED, held out to the public as a location for emergency care on an urgent basis without a scheduled appointment, and/or a facility that provided at least one-third of its outpatient visits for emergency care on an urgent basis without a scheduled appointment during the prior calendar year (*Medicare Claims Processing Manual,* Chapter 4, §160, 2015).

- Type B hospital ED visits, as defined by EMTALA, are billed using HCPCS Level II codes (G0380–G0384). A Type B ED is a dedicated ED that is not open 24 hours a day, 7 days a week (*Medicare Claims Processing Manual*, Chapter 4, §160, 2015).

CMS allows hospitals to establish their own internal system of assigning coding levels for the facility component of ED visits, as long as levels are reasonably related to the intensity of hospital resources utilized, the basis for the system is clear and well-documented, and the codes are applied consistently (72 *Fed. Reg.* 66580, 66805, 2007).

Hospitals may also bill for critical care services (CPT code 99291) instead of a clinic or emergency department visit code (HCPCS code G0463) when those criteria are met (*Medicare Claims Processing Manual*, Chapter 23, §20.7.6.3.2(C), 2015). In addition, when the guidelines are met, hospitals may bill for trauma activation services if the hospital is licensed or designated as a Level I–IV Trauma Center (*Medicare Claims Processing Manual*, Chapter 25, §75.4, 2015). Hospitals bill for other therapeutic and diagnostic services using the appropriate HCPCS or revenue code.

Facility component: Modifiers

Just like on the professional claim, the hospital should use the appropriate modifiers when billing the facility component of provider-based services (*Medicare Claims Processing Manual*, Chapter 4 §§20.6–20.6.11, 2015). For example, modifier -52 may be required on the UB-04 for diagnostic tests to indicate that these are split-billed (*Medicare Claims Processing Manual*, Chapter 4 §§20.6–20.6.6, 2015).

In order to track the volume and type of services furnished in provider-based departments, CMS created a modifier for hospital reporting of services performed in off-campus provider-based hospital departments; the -PO modifier (79 *Fed. Reg.* 66770, 66914, 2014; *Medicare Claims Processing Manual*, Chapter 4 §20.6.11, 2015). This is an informational modifier that should be used on the 837I (UB-04 claim) on each and every line item for the services performed in an off-campus provider-based department. The modifier should be placed after the other payment modifiers.

Use of the -PO modifier was voluntary beginning January 1, 2015. However, CMS mandated the modified as of January 1, 2016 (*Medicare Claims Processing Manual*, Chapter 4 §20.6.11, 2015).

This modifier should not be used on the claims for on-campus provider-based departments. In accordance with 79 *Fed. Reg.* 66770, 66914 (2014) and the *Medicare Claims Processing Manual*,

Chapter 4 §20.6.11 (2015), the -PO modifier should not be used for the following off-campus departments:

- Remote locations of a hospital defined at 42 *CFR* 412.65

- Satellite facilities of a hospital defined at 42 *CFR* 412.22(h)

- Services furnished in an emergency department

CMS stated in 79 *Fed. Reg.* 66770, 66914 (2014) that it implemented this -PO modifier to gather information related to the services furnished in off-campus provider-based departments, including the:

- Frequency of services at provider-based clinics

- Type of services provided

- Payment for those services

The hospital industry should expect that once claims are submitted for off-campus departments with the -PO modifier, CMS (or its MAC) will audit the hospital's use of that provider-based clinic. Specifically, hospitals should expect CMS to actively review claims to determine whether the hospital filed an 855A application and a provider-based attestation for those entities. If the hospital has failed to add the off-campus location to its 855A application (hence, to its Medicare certification) and is billing for that entity, CMS will likely soon come knocking on the hospital's door to demand evidence that the hospital is in compliance with the provider-based requirements.

Summary of New Provider-Based Coding Requirements

A summary of the requirements for the use of the new -PO modifier and POS codes is furnished in Figure 6.7.

Figure 6.7	Summary of Requirements for Modifier -PO and Place of Service Codes	
Requirements for Use of "-PO" Modifier and Place of Service (POS) Codes		
	Hospital Billing (837I)	Professional Billing (837B)
On-Campus Department	Do not use -PO modifier	POS 22
Off-Campus Department	Use -PO modifier	POS 22 through December 31, 2015 POS 19 effective January 1, 2016

Source: Gina M. Reese, Esq., RN, an instructor for HCPro's Medicare Boot Camp®—Hospital Version and Medicare Boot Camp®—Utilization Review Version. Reprinted with permission.

Medicare Cost-Sharing and Deductibles in Provider-Based Departments

In addition to the monthly premium for Part B services, Medicare beneficiaries are responsible for a small annual deductible. For example, the annual deductible for calendar year 2015 is $147 (79 *Fed. Reg.* 61314, 61317, 2014). This deductible is not affected by provider-based billing. However, there are some services that are not subject to the deductible or coinsurance, such as home health services, clinical diagnostic laboratory tests, vaccines, community healthcare services, and certain preventive services.

Medicare beneficiaries are also liable for a coinsurance or copayment equal to approximately 20% of the Medicare allowable amount for each covered Part B service. Notably, although the Medicare program states that this is a 20% coinsurance, the actual coinsurance for services ranges from 20% to approximately 40%. CMS is gradually reducing the coinsurance for all services to 20%, but this will take a period of time to accomplish (*Medicare Claims Processing Manual*, Chapter 4 §30, 2015). Medicare beneficiaries who receive medical services at freestanding physician offices should only incur liability for one copayment for the visit. This cost-sharing is based on the Medicare-allowed amount paid to the physician for these services. In other words, the beneficiary is liable for 20–40% of the MPFS amount for these services.

In contrast, patients who seek the exact same services in a provider-based department receive bills for two copayments—one from the physician for the professional component of the services and the other from the hospital for the facility component of the services. The total amount paid to the physician and the hospital by Medicare for these services is generally more than the amount that would have been paid for these services in the freestanding physician office. Therefore, the beneficiary's liability for these services is also generally higher than the cost-sharing he or she would have been subjected to for these services at a freestanding physician office. This increase is more obvious because the beneficiary receives two separate bills: one from the hospital and one from the physician.

There is an example of this differential in beneficiary liability in the scenario discussed in Figure 6.5. The figure reflects a clinic visit (99213 for professional billing, G0463 for hospital outpatient billing) with a separately identifiable surgical procedure (excision of a lesion, CPT code 11420).

In this example, the patient's copayment in the physician's office is $46.02 for the visit. In the hospital-based outpatient department, the patient owes a lower amount for the professional services ($32.48), but owes $94.97 in copayment for the facility component of the services, which is a total of $127.45, an increase of 277% in liability for the beneficiary in the hospital-based department for exactly the same services. For Medicare beneficiaries on fixed budgets (and practically anyone else), this is a significant hit to the bottom line.

CMS expressed this concern in regulations dealing with provider-based status:

> *"In many cases, there is also an increase in beneficiaries' out-of-pocket expenses compared to services furnished in a physician office. For example, when a beneficiary is treated in a physician office, the only payment made is Part B payment to the physician for his or her professional services, under the physician fee schedule. The single payment made under the physician fee schedule pays for the physician's work and includes a component for practice expense. The beneficiary's coinsurance is based on 20 percent of the physician fee schedule amount. However, if the same service is furnished in a hospital outpatient clinic, Medicare Part B payment for a facility fee is also made to the hospital, in addition to the physician's payment (which may include a smaller practice expense component). Thus, for the same visit, the beneficiary is also subject to the Part B coinsurance for the hospital's facility fee. Beneficiaries are responsible for coinsurance based on 20 percent of the hospital's charges (or, the applicable coinsurance amounts under the hospital outpatient PPS)."*

—63 *Fed. Reg.* 47552, 47588, 1998.

Medicare beneficiaries may not always understand the reason that they receive two bills instead of just one. It is also unlikely that they understand why they pay more for the services at hospital-based clinics, especially since provider-based clinics often appear to be nearly identical to freestanding physician offices, and there is no difference in the actual services they receive. In fact, Medicare beneficiaries have become increasingly vocal about the inequities they perceive in such a system, although it is clear that there is also a tremendous misunderstanding about the facility fee involved in such billing. In one recent article in the *LA Times*, the patient did not appear to even be able to get a straight answer about the $546 facility fee billed by the hospital for a knee injection apparently administered in a hospital-based clinic (Hospital Isn't Shy About Getting Its Take, 2014).

Based on this outrage, CMS became more and more concerned about ensuring that the higher payments to provider-based clinics are justified. CMS has even cited editorials and articles that discuss the patient's perspective on the receipt of two bills and higher liability they are facing in provider-based clinics, even from third-party payers other than Medicare (78 *Fed. Reg.* 43534, 43627, 2013). In the article cited by CMS, the critics included community leaders and even physicians who practice in the provider-based clinics (Why you might pay twice for one visit to a doctor, 2012; Rising hospital employment of physicians, 2011).

Beneficiaries are more likely to raise concerns about the increased copayment if a hospital has recently acquired a location that previously operated as a freestanding physician office. In those cases, the patients may have been paying a lower copayment for the same services, and then suddenly experience a huge increase in liability for the same services furnished by the same physician. If the hospital has always operated the provider-based clinic, it is considered the norm by their patients, and they are less likely to be disturbed by the amount of their liability. Hospitals may fail to educate patients as to increased requirements when a clinic is acquired. Hospitals want to keep the clinic the same as it was prior to the acquisition, and this may be a huge and costly mistake. Instead, the hospital should ensure that its patients are educated about the new billing practices that they will encounter with the transition of a freestanding clinic to a provider-based setting.

Auditing for Compliance and Common Pitfalls

7

Overview

The biggest mistake in provider-based billing would be to simply start adding the -PO modifier when billing for off-campus departments and assume that the other criteria are already met. A more prudent approach is to take everything you have learned and conduct an audit of the hospital-based departments to ensure that they meet CMS expectations for these locations. In this final chapter, we hope to offer some practical pointers to use in identifying some of the most common issues and errors in provider-based billing, as well some tips on auditing for compliance with these requirements.

Auditing for Compliance

From the prior chapters, you should have all of the information you need to audit for compliance with the provider-based billing requirements. However, at this point, you are probably feeling a little overwhelmed and wondering where to start. What you need is a tool to organize these criteria and focus your audit. You may have already started making lists of the requirements and have an idea how you best want to conduct this audit. In case you need some guidance, a sample checklist for compliance is included at the end of this chapter to assist in organizing the audit process (see Figure 7.1). Of course, this checklist is no substitute for legal advice, especially for complex organizations under joint ventures, management contracts, or other complicated structures. It is recommended that any audit of these situations be informed by legal counsel.

Auditing is a team sport

We started this book with the premise that you are reading this as a new revenue cycle director who was asked to ensure your facility is in compliance with the provider-based requirements. Well, doesn't it make sense for the billing director to audit this? Aren't these billing requirements?

Actually, that's the wrong approach. Auditing for these requirements is a team sport. Hopefully, you have seen by now that very few of the provider-based compliance requirements are strictly about how to bill for these services. Instead, the vast majority of these requirements are clinical, organizational, and operational in nature. Therefore, all of the hospital leadership and staff must be involved in compliance, from the frontline clinical staff, to the billing and coding staff, to the medical records department, to the executive suite, to the corporate board, and many staff members in between.

The first step in any compliance project this broad is to identify the necessary leaders for the team and others from whom input should be sought. As you review the prior chapters and the sample audit checklist at the end of this chapter (see Figure 7.1), you will see, at a minimum, that the following hospital and medical staff should be involved in this team effort, both to ensure compliance and to furnish documentation and information necessary to support auditing efforts:

- Governing body

- Executive leadership

- Chief compliance officer and departmental compliance officers

- Medical staff office and leadership

- Finance leadership, including those responsible for hospital cost-reporting

- Revenue cycle director

- Medical records/health information management leadership

- Administrator for the EHR

- Regulatory staff that manage licensing, accreditation, and certification applications/ submissions

- Directors of utilization management and performance improvement/quality management

- Director(s) of facility management

- Admitting/registration director

- Administration and medical directors of each provider-based department

- Managers of contracted services

- Coders/billers—both professional and facility billing

- Physicians and nursing staff

- Legal counsel, as necessary, especially if there are joint ventures or management contracts

Although the managers and directors of the actual provider-based departments are important to the auditing efforts, the actual work of reviewing compliance should not be left strictly in the hands of those managers. It is not wise to trust the objectivity of managers reviewing their own departments. This creates the classic scenario where the fox is guarding the henhouse. However, even if the managers could be objective, any audit completed by the managers of the provider-based department would be incomplete, since they are not able to effectively judge the integration of these departments into the operation of the main provider. As noted above, this can only be demonstrated and supported by the other departments and high-level executives at the main hospital.

What to audit

After identifying the compliance team, the next step is to define the size and shape of the playing field. Although leadership should be able to readily identify the scope and location of all of their own hospital operations, the reality is that they are often unable to accurately list all of the various hospital departments and the legal character of these services. For example, the chief executive officer may be able to recognize that the hospital is affiliated with a clinic down the street, but may not be able to correctly identify whether the services are furnished by hospital employees or under a management contract, or operate as a freestanding clinic. In fact, hospital executives may not even be able to correctly list all of the hospital operations. They may accurately identify large scale operations, but fail to remember all of the related services and departments. Even the lowly phlebotomy stations located in outlying buildings need to be mapped and reviewed. If the hospital does not know the details about the operations of its provider-based clinics, or fails to audit some of them, it is impossible to determine full compliance. Therefore, the first task in the audit is to create an accurate detailed list of the provider operations and actually map their physical locations.

This mapping exercise may be more difficult than it initially appears, because it is likely that no single staff member has access to all of the information necessary to ensure a complete list of the hospital outpatient services. The first stop should be the facilities manager or similar person who is responsible for maintaining the building plans. Hopefully these plans contain details about all of the hospital buildings, both on and off campus. However, many times these facility plans only include information about the buildings actually owned by the hospital and fail to include other locations leased by the hospital or operated under other types of arrangements. In addition, these facility maps may be outdated for various reasons, including rapid growth and recent acquisitions. The end result is that these maps may not be detailed, complete, or accurate enough to be the only source of information about the hospital facility services.

Another source of information for the mapping is the performance improvement, regulatory, and/or compliance leaders in charge of licensing, certification, and/or accreditation of the hospital services. This may include more than one person in larger and more complex hospital systems, which may have more than one accrediting and licensing agency (e.g., stroke, bariatric, psychiatric, other specialty services). These staff members are charged with furnishing lists of hospital services to regulatory agencies, which may be even more complete than the facility maps.

From this basic set of information, the team should develop both a physical map of the hospital facilities and a detailed laundry list of all of the hospital services, both on and off campus. The map should identify the main hospital buildings, which are contiguous to each other, the buildings and other locations situated within 250 yards of the main buildings, and clinical departments located more than 250 yards off the main hospital campus. The map should also include any satellite facilities and remote locations operated by the hospital. The list of hospital departments should capture the following:

- Name/type of service(s) furnished in each location

- The actual physical address of these locations

- Whether the building is owned or leased

- The name and contact information of the landlord of any leased locations

- Whether the location is on- or off-campus, and, if off-campus, the distance from the main campus

This is a good time to start gathering and organizing the big picture organizational documents from the main provider necessary to substantiate that the provider-based department is integrated with the main provider.

The last step in this first phase of the audit is an actual walk-through of all of the hospital facilities and locations to verify the actual street address and services furnished at each location. During the walk-through, auditing staff should not only update the map and list of services, but should also ask about any services/locations not already on the map and begin the next phase of the audit—the collection of documents and other information necessary to complete the provider-based audit checklist (see Figure 7.1). The mapping and verification process may be quick and simple or lengthy and complex, reflecting the relative simplicity or complexity of the hospital operations.

Auditing criteria

As detailed in the sample audit checklist found at the end of this chapter (see Figure 7.1), the hospital staff should audit for compliance with each requirement under the provider-based regulations. As the staff works through the checklist, evidence of compliance should be collected from the department and organized in a compliance folder or notebook to memorialize the results of the audit. At the completion of the audit, all of this evidence should be scanned into an electronic file and updated as necessary as an ongoing compliance record to be produced in case of an external governmental audit. In addition, if the provider is planning to submit an attestation for some or all of the provider-based departments, some of this documentation will need to be submitted with the attestation, and the remainder must be maintained in the hospital records as support for the attestation and any subsequent audits.

Common Pitfalls in Provider-Based Compliance

Auditing for some of the provider-based criteria is fairly straightforward, but there are some common mistakes that hospitals have made that will be discussed below.

Failure to map and account for all provider-based spaces

Some providers are organized in a very simplistic fashion and change very little over time. These providers will have less difficulty completing a provider-based audit. For example, a stand-alone hospital with very few hospital outpatient services is unlikely to have any difficulty listing its provider-based departments and auditing them for compliance in a fairly rapid fashion. However, most hospital organizations are much more complex and are busily integrating both horizontally and vertically. As noted in Chapter 1, physician practices are increasingly integrating with hospitals. In addition, hospitals are consolidating into chain organizations through ownership, joint ventures, and other legal structures. As a consequence, a single hospital may have hundreds of distinct outpatient services, satellite facilities, and/or remote locations. To add to the complexity, the list of services furnished in a single hospital may rapidly and dramatically change from one year to the next. Therefore, despite the hospital's best efforts, the staff may lose track of the location and number of services furnished by the hospital and, hence, may fail to ensure that these services are added to (and subtracted from) the hospital license and 855A in a timely fashion, and that new locations are in compliance with the Medicare provider-based criteria.

As noted in Chapter 3, two of the threshold requirements for ensuring compliance with the provider-based criteria are addition of the location to the hospital license and submission of a revised CMS 855A with the address of the new hospital department. In addition, these requirements are essential to at least reducing the penalty if the other requirements are not met. With the rapidly changing environment described above, it is easy to see how these basic require-ments could be missed.

Over and above the requirement to add any new provider-based location to the hospital license, there is also a requirement to report new service locations to the hospital's MAC within 90 days of the effective date of the change, regardless of whether the provider is going to file a provid-er-based attestation (42 *CFR* §424.520[b], 2011). Failure to report such changes within 90 days may result in the deactivation or revocation of the hospital's Medicare billing privileges. These changes must be made by filing a revised CMS 855A form with the hospital's MAC.

Because of the risks associated with billing incorrectly in provider-based spaces, as well as fail-ing to meet the CMS requirements to report revisions in service locations, hospitals should con-sider implementing a very rigorous process to manage any changes (additions or deletions) in hospital services (i.e., a change management process). This process would address various other concerns besides compliance with the provider-based criteria.

A mature change management process includes all important decision-makers and integrates a thorough approval and vetting of all new services and practice locations long prior to the actual acquisition of the service, construction of new buildings, or registration of any patients. Besides approval of the strategic plan and budget for the new service, the change management process should incorporate research into and compliance with regulatory requirements such as the pro-vider-based requirements. By combining all of these functions into one process, the hospital will be sure to bake compliance into the service and plan to set aside sufficient time to ensure that the location is not acquired and the service is not initiated until all of the required applications are submitted, and all compliance and regulatory approvals are received. A sample change man-agement checklist is included at the end of this chapter (see Figure 7.2).

Similarly, the change management process should also be utilized for any revisions in the nature or location of hospital services. For example, when a hospital physically moves the location of a clinical department or service, the change management team should approve the planned move, ensure that the new location meets all regulatory and other requirements, and submit any appli-cations for approval of this new location prior to the actual relocation of the department. These are considerations even when the hospital plans to terminate services or dispose of hospital buildings. Again, the change management decision-makers should ensure that the necessary changes are made to the hospital licenses, accreditation, and Medicare/Medicaid certification, and that any other regulatory requirements are met in an integrated fashion.

If this change management process is maintained in an ongoing fashion, there should be no need to perform periodic audits of compliance of the hospital services. Instead, compliance will be ensured as a required component of the strategic planning for all hospital operations. As a result, the hospital will always be prepared for an audit by the government and will not have to scramble to pull documents together at the last minute only to find that some important detail (like adding a department to the state license) has been overlooked.

Sharing space with a freestanding entity

As evidenced by multimillion dollar settlements with the OIG and CMS by hospitals in 2011, 2014, and 2015, one of the biggest pitfalls in meeting the provider-based requirements is when a provider-based department shares space with a distinct freestanding entity (Denial of Hospital Off-Site Location, 2011; Settlement Agreement Between United States of America and Our Lady of Lourdes Memorial Hospital, 2014; Provider-Based Rules Trigger, 2015). CMS has been warning hospitals about this issue for several years and has begun recouping money paid to provider-based departments that make this mistake. For example, in a letter dated July 22, 2011, CMS determined that an entity failed to qualify as a hospital-based department for an Indiana hospital because, among other things, the entity shared space with a freestanding facility (Denial of Hospital Off-Site Location, 2011). CMS stated that sharing space with a freestanding entity violated the provider-based criteria in the following ways:

- **Does not meet definition of department of a provider.** *"To the extent that a facility does not meet the definition of a department of a provider [under 42 CFR §413.65(a)(2)], the facility cannot have provider-based status as a department of a provider. A department of a provider requires sufficient separation from any other facility. Sufficiently separated space is indicated by such features as exclusive entrance, waiting, and registration areas, permanent walls, and a distinct suite designation recognized by the United States Postal Service if the hospital department does not occupy an entire building."*

  —Denial of Hospital Off-Site Location, 2011.

- **Does not meet hospital *CoPs*.** *"When a would-be hospital department shares space with freestanding offices, CMS must consider the entire space that contains the purported hospital department and the space's relationship to the hospital's CoPs at 42 CFR Part 485 Subpart F … CMS may consider a suite in a medical office building to be a singular component for compliance with the hospital CoPs … However, CMS cannot consider only portions of a singular component when determining if these criteria are met … A main provider hospital may not lease or otherwise obtain use of a portion of a singular component within that space. Certain features, such as shared entryways, interior hallways, bathroom facilities, treatment rooms, waiting rooms, and registration areas are all indications that a purported hospital space may instead be a part of a larger component. Building plans that do not clearly demarcate a purported hospital space as a distinct space is another possible indicator that the space is not a self-contained component. Rent that is paid to a tenant of a building* *rather than directly to the building owner or landlord may also be an indication that a space does not itself constitute a singular component."*

—*Denial of Hospital Off-Site Location*, 2011.

- **Promotes abusive practices.** *"Were CMS to permit hospitals to carve out spaces or services at freestanding facilities, hospitals and physicians would be able to make arrangements that would allow for the maximization of reimbursement for services depending on how certain services are reimbursed in certain settings."*

  — Denial of Hospital Off-Site Location, 2011.

- **Public awareness requirement not met.** *"[T]he public awareness requirement is not met to the extent that the singular component is held out as a freestanding supplier of services, even if it is also held out to the public as a furnisher of hospital services."*

  — Denial of Hospital Off-Site Location, 2011.

CMS increased enforcement of its prohibition on sharing of space in 2014 and 2015. As discussed in earlier chapters, in addition to the case described above, the OIG has sought millions in repayments based on violations of the provider-based requirement due to sharing of space with freestanding entities. There are not yet a lot of details publicly available about the details in these cases, but one hospital settled a provider-based billing case for $3.37 million and another hospital reportedly settled a very similar case for $2.63 million—both based on the fact that the hospitals shared space with freestanding facilities (Settlement Agreement Between United States of America and Our Lady of Lourdes Memorial Hospital, 2014; Provider-Based Rules Trigger, 2015).

Based on these cases, it is clear that CMS takes the issue of shared space seriously. Therefore, a hospital must ensure the following is true when conducting an audit:

- That hospital-based departments occupy an entire suite completely separate from any surrounding freestanding entities, including any entrances, hallways, and bathroom facilities
- That the rent for this location is paid to the building owner or landlord rather than to another tenant of the building
- That the freestanding entity does not borrow the space from the provider-based department during off-hours
- That the building plans completely support this separation

A walk-through of the hospital-based department both during the day and off-hours would be warranted to demonstrate that the space is not shared any time of the day or night.

Failure to meet hospital outpatient coverage requirements

There is an extensive list of coverage requirements that must be met to furnish outpatient services to Medicare beneficiaries, which we reviewed in some detail in Chapter 5. Hospitals may find that certain coverage requirements for therapeutic and diagnostic service are more difficult to meet than others, especially in off-campus provider-based departments. The following are some of the trickier issues that hospitals should audit more carefully in the process of monitoring for compliance in provider-based departments:

- **New therapeutic services without physician order or ongoing physician involvement.** A physician order is required to meet the Medicare coverage requirements, as detailed in Chapter 5. However, the nursing staff may not always obtain a physician's order to perform all of the therapeutic services furnished to Medicare beneficiaries. This is a common occurrence when nurses are treating patients under protocols for ongoing monitoring and treatment, where they may begin treatment of a new problem without first consulting with the physician and obtaining an order for the new services. For example, a nurse is furnishing treatment under the physician's orders for a wound on the foot for three months, then notices a new wound on the lower leg and begins the same treatment for that wound without contacting the physician and obtaining orders for the new wound treatment. While the nurse may be correct about the need for these services, proceeding with the treatment without the physician's order is not only a violation of the incident to physician order rule, but is also likely to be found a violation of the nurse's state license scope of practice. Both of these issues could cause Medicare to find that these services are not covered and that the provider-based department is out of compliance. Reimbursement for these services may therefore be considered an overpayment.

  Be mindful of this issue in particular when auditing compliance in provider-based departments where nurses treat patients over a long period of time for chronic conditions. As noted above, nurses treating patients with chronic illnesses under protocols for ongoing monitoring and treatment often begin treatment of a new problem without first consulting with the physician and obtaining an order for the new services. Besides creating a problem under the physician ordering rule, this violates the requirement that the physician have periodic involvement with the patient and personally see the patient at the beginning of any treatment plan. The hospital must ensure that the nurses send the patients back to the physician for an assessment of the new or worsening condition, which will likely result in new orders for that condition.

  In addition to auditing for therapeutic services performed without physician orders, consider establishing specific guidelines in chronic care clinics that require that:

  - Patients be referred for a physician visit with any new clinical problems

- Patients be required to be personally seen by the physician at intervals specified by the medical staff for their condition, and

- Orders for the ongoing treatment be reassessed during the physician assessment and renewed only if still medically necessary

In addition, nursing staff must be mindful of obtaining orders for any new services and documenting all patient contact with the physician to demonstrate the physician's ongoing oversight of the services.

- **Order by a physician with no hospital privileges.** As noted in Chapter 5, the physician or NPP ordering therapeutic services must have clinical privileges at the hospital. There is a particular scenario that may cause insidious problems with this requirement. A physician may see a patient in his or her freestanding physician office and order a service that needs to be performed in the hospital provider-based department, such as an infusion service or transfusion. If this physician does not have clinical privileges at the hospital, his or her order for the services is not sufficient to meet the order requirement under the incident to services. In this situation, the nursing staff is usually prohibited from accepting this order under the hospital's bylaws, rules, and regulations. The nursing staff may not pick up on this point and may perform these services, because they are ordered by a physician. However, acceptance of this order may lead Medicare to determine that the service is not covered, and acceptance of payment from Medicare for this service may be considered an overpayment.

This is an important point to audit in reviewing compliance with incident to requirements. In addition, the hospital may consider drafting a policy and procedure that requires nursing staff to check any new orders for services against a list of medical staff members and privileges to ensure that the order is from someone with clinical privileges at the hospital. There could be an automatic cross-check established within a hospital's EHR to ensure that the orders received are from physicians with hospital privileges.

- **Supervision of hospital outpatient therapeutic and diagnostic services.** There are many potential pitfalls with the requirement that hospital outpatient services be supervised at the appropriate level under the incident to coverage requirements, as detailed in Chapter 5. These requirements should be audited closely, since they are highly scrutinized by CMS.

One of the requirements under the supervision rule is that the supervising physician or NPP must be available throughout the performance of the procedure. This requirement seems self-explanatory and, on the surface, does not appear to be difficult to implement. However, the challenge is ensuring that the physician or NPP is actually available during all of the days of the week and hours of the day that the clinic furnishes services and does not disappear prior to the time the procedure is actually completed. For example, if a hospital-based clinic is open during the evening hours to accommodate patients who work during the day, the physician or NPP must also be available for those same hours. At times, the physician is available during the main portion of the procedures, but not available during the time that the patient is recovering after the procedure. Services that must be supervised include both the actual procedure and any pre- and post-procedure recovery. Any mismatch in schedules may cause problems with this requirement. Therefore, you must audit the schedule of the supervising physician or NPP to ensure that there is a one-to-one match with the hours the services are furnished.

Under the current supervision rules for hospital outpatient diagnostic and therapeutic services, there is no limitation on the location of the supervising physician per se. As long as the physician meets the other requirements listed above, including the mandate that the physician be immediately available, the supervising physician or NPP may be located in the actual department, on the hospital campus, or in nonhospital property close to the hospital. This includes any location in a building off campus that houses multiple provider-based departments. However, as a practical matter, it is hard to understand how a physician or NPP could be located as far as CMS states is possible for supervision of hospital departments (off the hospital campus or in or near medical office buildings) and still be immediately available as described by CMS. It seems nearly impossible for a physician to be potentially miles off campus and still respond without a lapse of time.

Many hospitals, especially small facilities, struggle to find enough physicians who agree to supervise the hospital outpatient services. These hospitals would like to believe that the answer lies in using the emergency room physicians to furnish this supervision, since they are required to stay on the hospital campus to treat patients in the emergency department. However, use of these physicians could be challenged, since they are often tied up treating other patients and are therefore unable to actually respond immediately.

To my knowledge, there have been no real tests of how CMS will enforce these requirements, but the hospital should carefully audit this requirement. If possible, the hospital should consider drafting policies and procedures that mandate that the supervising physician or NPP remain as close as possible to the hospital outpatient department and not be involved in complex procedures with other patients so that he or she remains immediately available to step in and perform as required. Preferably, supervising physicians should be directly assigned to the department, especially in busy off-campus provider-based departments.

In addition to the difficulties with the immediate availability of the supervising physician or NPP, hospitals often find it hard to demonstrate which physician is supervising the provider-based department at any one time. There are various methods of verifying that a supervising physician is present at a designated time, including, but not limited to:

- Maintaining a schedule of supervising physicians

- Instructing the nursing staff to document the name of the supervising physician in the encounter note

- Instructing the nursing staff to document the encounter in an electronic system that links the supervising physician with the billing system

Whichever method is selected, the hospital must perform an audit which verifies that the supervising physician documented in the system or on the schedule was actually available (e.g., was not on vacation, did not call in sick). In addition, it is useful to do a walk-through audit of the provider-based clinics, especially those located off-campus. During this audit, the auditor may want to ask the nursing staff for the identity of the supervising physician or NPP, and then call that physician or NPP to determine whether he or she can respond quickly enough to support the theory that this supervisor is actually immediately available, as required.

Use of the correct POS code on physician billing for provider-based services

As noted in earlier chapters, one of the basic requirements for compliance with provider-based billing is that the professional claims must be submitted on the CMS 1500 form using the POS for hospital outpatient services. The POS code 22 must be used until the end of 2015. Effective January 1, 2016, POS code 22 will continue to be used for services furnished in on-campus hospital outpatient departments, but POS code 19 must be used when billing for services furnished in off-campus hospital departments. As detailed in Chapter 6, the hospital's MAC and the OIG are easily able to audit whether the hospital-based physicians are correctly billing using the POS for provider-based locations. In fact, the OIG is carefully monitoring this issue, resulting in recoupment of overpayments made to physicians as the result of the use of the incorrect POS code.

The executive leadership may not believe that it is the hospital's responsibility to ensure that the physician claims contain the correct POS coding for hospital-based outpatient departments (POS code 22). However, if the professional claims for services furnished in a provider-based department are generated with the incorrect POS code, this affects both the physician and the hospital. The physician may face recoupment of an overpayment (and possibly other penalties), but the hospital may also be found out of compliance with the provider-based requirements for that clinic under 42 *CFR* §413.65(g)(2) (2011). In fact, CMS has expressly stated that both the physician and the hospital may be held responsible for insuring that physicians and NPPs are billing correctly for hospital-based services:

> *"Physicians who practice in hospitals, including off-site departments, do so under privileges granted by the hospitals. Thus, we believe the hospital has a role in ensuring proper billing."*

> —65 *Fed. Reg.* 18434, 18519, 2000.

Because of the high risk of noncompliance, a hospital operating a provider-based clinic must work closely with the entity that is generating the claims for the professional services furnished in that clinic to ensure that the POS code on those claims is 22, rather than 11.

In addition to concerns about the POS codes, there could also be problems with the professional claim if line items are included for the facility services furnished by the hospital outpatient department. As detailed in Chapter 6, these facility services must instead be billed by the hospital on the hospital claim. For example, if a diagnostic service is furnished in a hospital-based radiology department, and the interpretation is performed by a hospital-based physician, the professional claim may include only the professional component of the service and may not include the facility component of that service. If the professional claim also includes the facility component, this constitutes double billing for that service and may create doubt that the services were furnished in a provider-based department instead of a freestanding facility.

Given that the correct use of POS codes is one of the most readily audited requirements, this should also be one of the main criteria that hospitals audit on an ongoing basis if at all possible. Of course, if the professional services are billed by an agency that is distinct from the hospital billing services, auditing for this requirement is automatically more complex. Therefore, it is in the hospital's best interest to become as involved as possible in billing for hospital-based physicians. At minimum, the hospital should consider sending annual letters to the physician billing service reminding them about the appropriate POS code for the hospital-based locations. Ideally, the hospital will actually contract to act as the billing agent for the physicians who furnish services in the hospital-based clinics. This gives the hospital more oversight and control of the professional claims and ensures better compliance with the provider-based requirements. The hospital must determine whether this means that it will prepare claims for these physicians just for services provided in the provider-based department versus billing for services furnished at all locations, including those outside of the hospital at freestanding facilities.

Figure 7.1	Checklist for Audit of Provider-Based Departments		
Provider-Based Department Info and CMS Criteria From 42 *CFR* 413.65		Dept. _____	Dept. _____
Department Demographics			
1	Department name.		
2	Physical address. Attach map of location and building plan for location.		
3	Type of services furnished.		
4	Furnishes inpatient or outpatient services (or both)? Explain.		
5	Space leased or owned by main hospital? If owned, attach any ownership documents.		

Figure 7.1	Checklist for Audit of Provider-Based Departments (cont.)		
\#	Provider-Based Department Info and CMS Criteria From 42 *CFR* 413.65	Dept. _____	Dept. _____
6	If space is leased, list landlord and attach rental/lease contract.		
7	Distance from main hospital campus. Describe location, determination as to main hospital campus, and basis for determination of distance from that location. Attach map and any evidence used to make determination about distance.		
8	Name of medical director at location.		
9	Number and type of employees at location.		
10	Name/title of department administrator/director at location.		
11	Number of years and dates in operation.		
12	Does this department share space with another entity? If so, is it shared with hospital-based entity or nonhospital-based entity? Does the space overlap? Describe in detail and attach any pertinent information.		
13	Are any of the department's services furnished under agreement with another entity (e.g., management agreement or "under arrangements" agreement)? If so, with whom and describe. Attach agreement.		
14	Meets definition of "satellite facility" (provides inpatient services in a building also used by another hospital, or in one or more entire buildings located on the same campus as buildings used by another hospital)? Explain.		
15	Meets definition of remote facility (furnishes inpatient hospital services in another location under name, ownership, and control of the main hospital)? Explain.		
16	Who prepares the claims for the services from this location? Are the claims prepared by billers in the main hospital, contracted billing agency, or other? Explain in detail.		
17	Who employs the nonphysician staff in this department?		
18	Has the main provider filed a provider-based attestation for this department? If yes, list date(s) of attestation and attach attestation(s).		

Figure 7.1	Checklist for Audit of Provider-Based Departments (cont.)		
	Provider-Based Department Info and CMS Criteria From 42 *CFR* 413.65	Dept. _____	Dept. _____
	**Is This Location Exempt From Provider-Based Requirements?**
AA	Does this location furnish billable clinical services? If no, then explain and STOP—do not complete assessment (not required to meet provider-based requirements). If yes, proceed with remainder of assessment.		
BB	Does this location have a separate Medicare provider number (e.g., hospice, home health agency, ambulatory surgical center, skilled nursing facility)? If yes, explain and STOP–do not complete assessment (not required to meet provider-based requirements). If no, proceed with remainder of assessment.		
CC	Are the services furnished in this location billed under the hospital's provider number and name? If yes, proceed with assessment. If no, explain the billing in detail and STOP here—this is a freestanding entity, not a provider-based department.		
DD	Are all of the services furnished in this location provided by another entity "under arrangements?" If yes, explain, attach agreement, and STOP—do not complete assessment (not required to meet provider-based requirements). If no, proceed with assessment.		
	**All Provider-Based Departments, Regardless of Location, Must Meet the Following Requirements a–ab (any "no" answers require remediation).**
a	Is this location listed on the main hospital's state license (unless not allowed under state law, then enter "NA" and explain)? If listed on hospital's license, attach hospital license.		
b	Is this location listed as a hospital location on CMS 855A filed with Medicare Administrative Contractor? If yes, then attach 855A or other documentation that supports this conclusion.		
c	Is this location listed as a hospital department on the hospital organizational chart? If yes, attach organizational chart.		
d	Does the administrative manager of this department report up through the main hospital management structure? If yes, attach organizational chart or other evidence.		

Figure 7.1	Checklist for Audit of Provider-Based Departments (cont.)		
\multicolumn{2}{c}{Provider-Based Department Info and CMS Criteria From 42 *CFR* 413.65}	Dept. _____	Dept. _____
e	Do all professional staff (physicians and non-physician practitioners) who furnish services at this location have clinical privileges at the main provider? If yes, attach documents supporting this conclusion.		
f	Does the medical director for this location report to the hospital's medical director/chief medical officer? If yes, attach organizational chart or other documentation supporting this conclusion.		
g	Do the hospital medical staff committees supervise medical services at this location? If yes, attach documentation supporting this conclusion.		
h	Do the hospital commitees monitor/oversee the facility services at this location, including utilization management and PI/QA? If yes, attach documentation.		
i	Is this department under the same bylaws and policies and procedures as the main provider? If yes, attach evidence.		
j	Are the medical records at this location integrated with the hospital medical records (e.g., integrated electronic health record, medical records master patient index, or health information management retrievable cross reference to department records)? If yes, attach documentation supporting this conclusion.		
k	Do the outpatients at this location have access to services at the main hospital? If yes, explain conclusion, such as evidence of referrals of patients to main hospital.		
l	Is the cost center for this location found on the hospital general ledger, trial balance, and other financial reporting? If yes, attach examples.		
m	Is this location reported on hospital cost report? If yes, attach examples.		
n	Do this location's expense and revenue roll up to the main hospital's income statement and balance sheet? If yes, attach examples.		
o	Are this department's statistics and financials included in the main hospital's annual Medicare and Medicaid cost report?		

Figure 7.1	Checklist for Audit of Provider-Based Departments (cont.)		
	Provider-Based Department Info and CMS Criteria From 42 _CFR_ 413.65	Dept. _____	Dept. _____
p	Is this location held out to the public as part of the hospital on the hospital's website, public advertising, and all other public documents? If yes, attach examples.		
q	Do the department's signage, letterhead, and advertising hold the location out as part of the main hospital? If yes, attach examples.		
r	Does the reception staff at this location answer the phone and greet patients with a greeting signifying the department is part of the main hospital?		
s	Does the hospital phone book and internal and website listings include this department as part of the main hospital? If yes, attach examples.		
t	Does this location meet all hospital _Conditions of Participation_, including life safety codes provisions? If yes, attach survey report showing that this location has been surveyed by outside surveyors or as part of an internal hospital mock survey.		
u	Does the hospital ensure that services furnished at this location comply with the three-day payment window for Medicare beneficiaries (i.e., specified services provided up to three days before inpatient admission are included on inpatient claim) and one-day payment window for Medicaid patients? If yes, attach policies and procedures or other documentation to support this conclusion.		
v	Are all patients at this location registered as outpatients of the main hospital? If yes, attach sample claims or other documentation showing evidence of this.		
w	Does this location comply with EMTALA requirements (applies to on-campus departments and off-campus dedicated emergency departments)? If off-campus and not a dedicated emergency department, enter "NA." If yes, attach evidence of emergency log, policies and procedures, and other evidence of compliance.		

Figure 7.1	Checklist for Audit of Provider-Based Departments (cont.)		
	Provider-Based Department Info and CMS Criteria From 42 *CFR* 413.65	Dept. _____	Dept. _____
x	Are the professional services furnished at this location billed using the place of service code for hospital outpatient services ("22" for all services through December 31, 2015; effective January 1, 2016, "22" for on-campus departments, and "19" for off-campus departments)? If yes, attach sample of claims and P&P supporting this conclusion.		
y	Do the professionals at this location comply with nondiscrimination provisions? If yes, attach P&P and any other evidence supporting this conclusion.		
z	Do the services at this location comply with Medicare coverage rules, including the "incident to" requirements for outpatient services, for the services furnished in this location? If yes, attach policies and procedures and any other evidence supporting this conclusion.		
aa	If the main provider is a nonprofit organization, does this department follow the main provider's financial assistance and 501(r) requirements? If yes, attach evidence.		
ab	If the location is operated under a joint venture with the main provider, is the location at least partially owned by one of the providers, located on the campus of the main provider who is a partial owner, and meets the provider-based requirements for that same provider? If so, attach evidence of meeting these requirements and attach the joint venture agreement.		
	If Department Is Off-Campus (Located More Than 250 Yards Away From Main Hospital Campus), the Department Must Also Meet the Following Requirements A–M (any "no" answers require remediation).		
A	Is this department located within 35 miles of main hospital campus or, if not, does it meet one of the exceptions to this location requirement, such as a high degree of integration due to common patients between department and hospital (see 42 *CFR* 413.65[e][3])? If yes, attach map of location of department or evidence that it meets one of the other exceptions.		

Figure 7.1	Checklist for Audit of Provider-Based Departments (cont.)		
	Provider-Based Department Info and CMS Criteria From 42 *CFR* 413.65	Dept. _____	Dept. _____
B	Is the department located in same state as the main hospital (or in adjacent states only if allowed by state law)? If yes, attach map of locations.		
C	Is this location 100% owned by hospital? If yes, attach documentation of ownership.		
D	Is this location accountable to the same governing body as the main hospital? If yes, attach documentation supporting this conclusion.		
E	Does the location furnish a notice to its patients re: additional copayment for facility billing (see 42 *CFR* 413.65(g)(7)? If yes, attach examples of notice(s).		
F	Does the main hospital have final approval over this department's administrative decisions, personnel actions, personnel policies, contracts with outside parties, and medical staff appointments? If yes, attach examples.		
G	Are the services from this department billed through same billing system as other hospital services? If yes, attach evidence.		
H	Is the payroll for the employees of this department paid through the main hospital payroll system? If yes, attach evidence.		
I	Are the supplies, drugs, and other purchases for this department made through the same place and follow the systems and procedures for the main hospital? If yes, attach evidence.		
J	Are the human resource services, benefit package, and salary structure for this department's personnel furnished through the same department as the main provider? If yes, attach evidence.		
K	Is this location directly supervised by the main hospital and under the same frequency, intensity, and level of accountability to the main provider as any other hospital department? If yes, attach support for this conclusion.		
L	If this location is under a management contract, is the contract under the name of the main hospital and not a parent entity? Attach management contract.		

Figure 7.1	Checklist for Audit of Provider-Based Departments (cont.)

	Provider-Based Department Info and CMS Criteria From 42 *CFR* 413.65	Dept. _____	Dept. _____
M	If the location is under a management contract, does the main provider employ the staff at this location (except for management staff or physician/nonphysician practitioners), or does the same organization employ the staff both at the main provider and this location? If yes, attach the management agreement and evidence of the employment of the staff.		

Disclaimer: This is provided as a summary resource and does not substitute for qualified healthcare legal counsel review of appropriateness of provider-based status of each location.

*Source: **Gina M. Reese, Esq., RN,** an instructor for HCPro's Medicare Boot Camp®—Hospital Version and Medicare Boot Camp®— Utilization Review Version. Reprinted with permission.*

Figure 7.2	Hospital XYZ Change Management Request Form

Change Request #:_____

Instructions: Must be completed for any addition, revision, or deletion in clinical hospital services. Submitter completes Section A (General Information) for all submissions. Submitter also completes one of the following: Part B for request to add services/locations/departments; Part C for request for revision in services/locations/departments, including change in type of services, change of address; Part D for request for deletion or closure of services/locations/departments.
Change Management Committee: Based on submitted information, collect other information as necessary to ensure that all appropriate regulatory, information technology, financial, and other requirements are met for proposed revision.

Part A: General Information	
Name of submitter	
Type of submission (check one).	Addition/new clinical service:
	Revision in existing clinical service:
	Deletion of existing clinical service:
Date submitted.	
Brief summary of proposed change.	
Proposed effective date of change.	
Sponsors of proposed change: List committees, executives, physicians, or others backing the proposal.	
Part B: Addition of Services - Describe Proposed New Clinical Services in Detail Below	
Type of services (e.g., dialysis, infusion).	
Department name.	

Figure 7.2	Hospital XYZ Change Management Request Form (cont.)	
Reason for change. Describe in detail if change is proposed to meet financial, clinical care, regulatory, or other need/requirements.		
Physical address. Attach map of location and building plan for location.		
Furnishes inpatient or outpatient services? Or both? Explain.		
Space leased or owned by main hospital? If owned, attach any ownership documents.		
If leased, list landlord and attach rental/lease contract.		
Distance from main hospital campus. Describe location, determination as to main hospital campus, and basis for determination of distance from that location. Attach map and any evidence used to make determination about distance.		
Name of medical director at location.		
Number and type of employees at location.		
Name/title of department administrator/director at location.		
Will this department share space with another entity? If so, shared with hospital-based entity or nonhospital-based entity? Does the space overlap? Describe in detail and attach any pertinent information.		
Are any of the department's services furnished under agreement with another entity (e.g., management agreement or "under arrangements" agreement)? If so, with whom and describe. Attach agreement.		
Meets definition of "satellite facility" (provides inpatient services in a building also used by another hospital, or in one or more entire buildings located on the same campus as buildings used by another hospital)? Explain.		
Meets definition of "remote facility" (furnishes inpatient hospital services in another location under name, ownership and control of the main hospital)? Explain.		
Who prepares the claims for the services from this location? Prepared by billers in main hospital? Or contracted billing agency? Or other? Explain in detail.		
Who employs the nonphysician staff in this department?		
Is a state license required for this location? If so, attach the application and list lead time for approval.		

Figure 7.2	Hospital XYZ Change Management Request Form (cont.)	
Must this service be added to the Medicare 855A/ certification? If so, attach form and list lead time for approval.		
Does this service require any special certification, accreditation, or any other special approval? If so, attach required form and list lead time for approval.		
Part C: Revision of Services - Describe Proposed Revision in Clinical Services in Detail Below		
Type of services (e.g., dialysis, infusion).		
Department name.		
Furnishes inpatient or outpatient services? Or both? Explain.		
Reason for change: Describe in detail if change is proposed to meet financial, clinical care, regulatory, or other need/requirements.		
Describe proposed change in detail (e.g., change in location, services).		
If relocation, list current and proposed physical address. Attach map of location and building plan for location.		
Space leased or owned by main hospital? If owned, attach any ownership documents.		
If leased, list landlord and attach rental/lease contract.		
Distance from main hospital campus. Describe location, determination as to main hospital campus, and basis for determination of distance from that location. Attach map and any evidence used to make determination about distance.		
Does the change require regulatory approval? If so, attach application for change and list lead time for approval.		
Part D: Deletion of Services - Describe Proposed Deletion of Clinical Services in Detail Below		
Type of services (e.g., dialysis, infusion).		
Department name.		
Furnishes inpatient or outpatient services? Or both? Explain.		
Reason for change: Describe in detail if change is proposed to meet financial, clinical care, regulatory, or other need/requirements.		
Describe proposed change in detail (e.g., change in location, services).		

Figure 7.2	Hospital XYZ Change Management Request Form (cont.)	
Does the change require regulatory approval? If so, attach application for change and list lead time for approval.		
APPROVAL OF PROPOSED CHANGE IN CLINICAL SERVICES		
Approving department	Signature and date	
Director of department		
Head of change management committee		
Compliance officer		
Chief financial officer		
Chief executive officer		
[other approvals as necessary depending on type of proposed revision]		
Disclaimer: This is provided as a summary resource and does not substitute for qualified healthcare legal counsel review of addition, revision, or deletion of clinical services, departments, or locations.		

Source: **Gina M. Reese, Esq., RN,** an instructor for HCPro's Medicare Boot Camp®—Hospital Version and Medicare Boot Camp®—Utilization Review Version. Reprinted with permission.

References

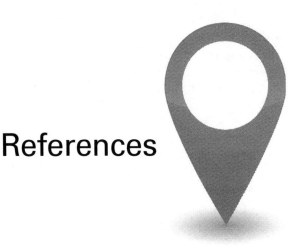

31 *USC* §§3729–3733. (2011). Retrieved August 10, 2015, from *www.gpo.gov/fdsys/pkg/USCODE-2011-title31/pdf/USCODE-2011-title31-subtitleIII-chap37-subchapIII-sec3729.pdf.*

42 *CFR* §405.2402 – Basic requirements. (2011). Retrieved August 10, 2015, from *www.gpo.gov/fdsys/granule/CFR-2011-title42-vol2/CFR-2011-title42-vol2-sec405-2402.*

42 *CFR* §405.2462 - Payment for rural health clinic and Federally qualified health center services. (2006). Retrieved August 10, 2015, from *www.gpo.gov/fdsys/granule/CFR-2011-title42-vol2/CFR-2011-title 42-vol2-sec405-2462.*

42 *CFR* §§405.2411–405.2417 - Scope of benefits. (2011). Retrieved August 10, 2015, from *www.gpo.gov/fdsys/search/pagedetails.action;jsessionid=sNzvVkQLmfRTx2YQ7YLy6DFKvwBT2BqBKt54LLqtTSqwjz GvdJJ2!-460559239!-514352434?collectionCode=CFR&searchPath=Title+42%2FChapter+IV%2F Subchapter+B%2FPart+405%2FSubpart+U&granuleId=CFR-2011-title42-vol2-sec405-2411&packageId= CFR-2011-title42-vol2&oldPath=Title+42%2FChapter+IV%2FSubchapter+B%2FPart+405%2FSubpart+X %2FSection+405.2411&fromPageDetails=true&collapse=true&ycord=800.*

42 *CFR* §409.16 - Other diagnostic or therapeutic services. (2011). Retrieved August 10, 2015, from *www.gpo.gov/fdsys/granule/CFR-2011-title42-vol2/CFR-2011-title42-vol2-sec409-16.*

42 *CFR* §409.3 - Definitions. (2011). Retrieved August 10, 2015, from *www.gpo.gov/fdsys/granule/CFR-1996-title42-vol2/CFR-1996-title42-vol2-sec409-3/content-detail.html.*

42 *CFR* §409.41 - Requirement for payment. (2011). Retrieved August 10, 2015, from *www.gpo.gov/fdsys/granule/CFR-2011-title42-vol2/CFR-2011-title42-vol2-sec409-41.*

42 *CFR* §410.15 - Annual wellness visits providing Personalized Prevention Plan Services: Conditions for and limitations on coverage. (2011). Retrieved August 10, 2015, from *www.gpo.gov/fdsys/granule/CFR-2011-title42-vol2/CFR-2011-title42-vol2-sec410-15.*

42 *CFR* §410.16 - Initial preventive physical examination: Conditions for and limitations on coverage. (2011). Retrieved August 10, 2015, from *www.gpo.gov/fdsys/pkg/CFR-2011-title42-vol2/pdf/CFR-2011-title42-vol2-sec410-16.pdf.*

42 *CFR* §410.17 - Cardiovascular disease screening tests. (2011). Retrieved August 10, 2015, from *www.gpo.gov/fdsys/granule/CFR-2011-title42-vol2/CFR-2011-title42-vol2-sec410-17.*

42 *CFR* §410.18 - Diabetes screening tests. (2011). Retrieved August 10, 2015, from *www.gpo.gov/fdsys/granule/CFR-2011-title42-vol2/CFR-2011-title42-vol2-sec410-18.*

42 *CFR* §410.19 - Ultrasound screening for abdominal aortic aneurysms: Condition for and limitation on coverage. (2011). Retrieved August 10, 2015, from *www.gpo.gov/fdsys/granule/CFR-2011-title42-vol2/ CFR-2011-title42-vol2-sec410-19.*

References

42 *CFR* §410.2 - Definitions. (2004). Retrieved August 10, 2015, from *www.gpo.gov/fdsys/granule/ CFR-2004-title42-vol2/CFR-2004-title42-vol2-sec410-2.*

42 *CFR* §410.27 - Outpatient hospital or CAH services and supplies incident to a physician or nonphysician practitioner service: Conditions. (2011). Retrieved August 10, 2015, from *www.gpo.gov/fdsys/granule/ CFR-2011-title42-vol2/CFR-2011-title42-vol2-sec410-27.*

42 *CFR* §410.28 - Hospital or CAH diagnostic services furnished to outpatients: Conditions. (2011). Retrieved August 10, 2015, from *www.gpo.gov/fdsys/pkg/CFR-2011-title42-vol2/pdf/CFR-2011-title42-vol2-sec410-28. pdf.*

42 *CFR* §410.31 - Bone mass measurement: Conditions for coverage and frequency standards. (2011). Retrieved August 10, 2015, from *www.gpo.gov/fdsys/pkg/CFR-2011-title42-vol2/pdf/CFR-2011-title42-vol2- sec410-31.pdf.*

42 *CFR* 410.32 - Diagnostic x-ray tests, diagnostic laboratory tests, and other diagnostic tests: Conditions. (2011). Retrieved August 10, 2015, from *www.gpo.gov/fdsys/granule/CFR-2011-title42-vol2/ CFR-2011-title42- vol2-sec410-32.*

42 *CFR* §410.33 - Independent diagnostic testing facility. (2011). Retrieved August 10, 2015, from *www.gpo. gov/fdsys/pkg/CFR-2011-title42-vol2/pdf/CFR-2011-title42-vol2-sec410-33.pdf.*

42 *CFR* §410.34 - Mammography services: Conditions for and limitations on coverage. (2011). Retrieved August 10, 2015, from *www.gpo.gov/fdsys/granule/CFR-2011-title42-vol2/CFR-2011-title42-vol2-sec410-34.*

42 *CFR* §410.36 - Medical supplies, appliances, and devices: Scope. (2011). Retrieved August 10, 2015, from *www.gpo.gov/fdsys/granule/CFR-2011-title42-vol2/CFR-2011-title42-vol2-sec410-36.*

42 *CFR* §410.37 - Colorectal cancer screening tests: Conditions for and limitations on coverage. (2011). Retrieved August 10, 2015, from *www.gpo.gov/fdsys/pkg/CFR-2011-title42-vol2/pdf/CFR-2011-title42-vol2- sec410-37.pdf.*

42 *CFR* §410.38 - Durable medical equipment: Scope and conditions. (2010). Retrieved August 10, 2015, from *www.gpo.gov/fdsys/granule/CFR-2010-title42-vol2/CFR-2010-title42-vol2-sec410-38.*

42 *CFR* §410.39 - Prostate cancer screening tests: Conditions for and limitations on coverage. (2011). Retrieved August 10, 2015, from *www.gpo.gov/fdsys/granule/CFR-2011-title42-vol2/CFR-2011-title42-vol2- sec 410-39.*

42 *CFR* §410.40 - Coverage of ambulance services. (2010). Retrieved August 10, 2015, from *www.gpo.gov/ fdsys/granule/CFR-2010-title42-vol2/CFR-2010-title42-vol2-sec410-40.*

42 *CFR* §410.41 - Requirements for ambulance suppliers. (2011). Retrieved August 10, 2015, from *www.gpo. gov/fdsys/granule/CFR-2011-title42-vol2/CFR-2011-title42-vol2-sec410-41.*

42 *CFR* §410.43 - Partial hospitalization services: Conditions and exclusions. (2011). Retrieved August 10, 2015, from *www.gpo.gov/fdsys/granule/CFR-2011-title42-vol2/CFR-2011-title42-vol2-sec410-43.*

42 *CFR* §410.47 - Pulmonary rehabilitation program: Conditions for coverage. (2010). Retrieved August 10, 2015, from *www.gpo.gov/fdsys/granule/CFR-2010-title42-vol2/CFR-2010-title42-vol2-sec410-47.*

42 *CFR* §410.48 - Kidney disease education services. (2011). Retrieved August 10, 2015, from *www.gpo.gov/ fdsys/granule/CFR-2011-title42-vol2/CFR-2011-title42-vol2-sec410-48.*

42 *CFR* §410.49 - Cardiac rehabilitation program and intensive cardiac rehabilitation program: Conditions of coverage. (2009). Retrieved August 10, 2015, from *www.gpo.gov/fdsys/granule/CFR-2011-title42-vol2/ CFR-2011-title42-vol2-sec410-49.*

 © 2015 HCPro

42 *CFR* §410.50 - Institutional dialysis services and supplies: Scope and conditions. (2011). Retrieved August 10, 2015, from *www.gpo.gov/fdsys/granule/CFR-2011-title42-vol2/CFR-2011-title42-vol2-sec410-50*.

42 *CFR* §410.56 - Screening pelvic examinations. (2011). Retrieved August 10, 2015, from *www.gpo.gov/fdsys/granule/CFR-2011-title42-vol2/CFR-2011-title42-vol2-sec410-56*.

42 *CFR* §410.57 - Pneumococcal vaccine and flu vaccine. (2011). Retrieved August 10, 2015, from *www.gpo.gov/fdsys/granule/CFR-2011-title42-vol2/CFR-2011-title42-vol2-sec410-57*.

42 *CFR* §410.59 - Outpatient occupational therapy services: Conditions. (2011). Retrieved August 10, 2015, from *www.gpo.gov/fdsys/granule/CFR-2011-title42-vol2/CFR-2011-title42-vol2-sec410-59*.

42 *CFR* §410.60 - Outpatient physical therapy services: Conditions. (2011). Retrieved August 10, 2015, from *www.gpo.gov/fdsys/granule/CFR-2011-title42-vol2/CFR-2011-title42-vol2-sec410-60*.

42 *CFR* §410.60(e) - Outpatient physical therapy services: Conditions. (2011). Retrieved August 10, 2015, from *www.gpo.gov/fdsys/granule/CFR-2011-title42-vol2/CFR-2011-title42-vol2-sec410-60*.

42 *CFR* §410.62 - Outpatient speech-language pathology services: Conditions and exclusions. (2011). Retrieved August 10, 2015, from *www.gpo.gov/fdsys/granule/CFR-2011-title42-vol2/CFR-2011-title42-vol2-sec 410- 62*.

42 *CFR* §410.63 - Hepatitis B vaccine and blood clotting factors: Conditions. (2011). Retrieved August 10, 2015, from *www.gpo.gov/fdsys/granule/CFR-2011-title42-vol2/CFR-2011-title42-vol2-sec410-63*.

42 *CFR* §410.75 - Nurse practitioners' services. (2011). Retrieved August 10, 2015, from *www.gpo.gov/fdsys/pkg/CFR-2011-title42-vol2/pdf/CFR-2011-title42-vol2-sec410-75.pdf*.

42 *CFR* §410.78 - Telehealth services. (2011). Retrieved August 10, 2015, from *www.gpo.gov/fdsys/granule/CFR-2011-title42-vol2/CFR-2011-title42-vol2-sec410-78*.

42 *CFR* §412.106(c)(2) - Special treatment: Hospitals that serve a disproportionate share of low-income patients. (2010). Retrieved August 10, 2015, from *www.gpo.gov/fdsys/pkg/CFR-2010-title42-vol2/pdf/CFR-2010-title42-vol2 sec412-106.pdf*.

42 *CFR* §412.2(c)(5) - Basis of payment. (2011). Retrieved August 10, 2015, from *www.gpo.gov/fdsys/pkg/CFR-2011-title42-vol2/pdf/CFR-2011-title42-vol2-sec412-2.pdf*.

42 *CFR* §412.22 - Excluded hospitals and hospital units: General rules. (2011). Retrieved August 10, 2015, from *www.gpo.gov/fdsys/granule/CFR-2011-title42-vol2/CFR-2011-title42-vol2-sec412-22*.

42 *CFR* §412.25 - Excluded hospital units: Common requirements. (2010). Retrieved August 10, 2015, from *www.gpo.gov/fdsys/granule/CFR-2010-title42-vol2/CFR-2010-title42-vol2-sec412-25*.

42 *CFR* 412.50(c) - Furnishing of inpatient hospital services directly or under arrangements. (2011). Retrieved August 10, 2015, from *www.gpo.gov/fdsys/granule/CFR-2011-title42-vol2/CFR-2011-title42-vol2-sec412-50*.

42 *CFR* 412.622(a)(3) – Basis of Payment. (2011). Retrieved August 10, 2015, from *www.gpo.gov/fdsys/pkg/CFR-2011-title42-vol2/pdf/CFR-2011-title42-vol2-sec412-622.pdf*.

42 *CFR* Part 413, Subpart J - Scope of benefits. (2011). Retrieved August 10, 2015, from *www.gpo.gov/fdsys/search/pagedetails.action?collectionCode=CFR&searchPath=Title+42%2FChapter+IV%2FSubchapter+B%2FPart+413%2FSubpart+J&granuleId=CFR-2011-title42-vol2-sec405-2411&packageId=CFR-2011-title42-vol2&oldPath=Title+42%2FChapter+IV%2FSubchapter+B%2FPart+413&fromPageDetails=true&collapse=true&ycord=1010.6666666666666*.

References

42 *CFR* §413.65 - Requirements for a determination that a facility or an organization has provider-based status. (2011). Retrieved August 10, 2015, from *www.gpo.gov/fdsys/granule/CFR-2011-title42-vol2/CFR-2011-title42 vol2-sec 413-65.*

42 *CFR* §414.1 et seq., Basis and scope. (2015). Retrieved August 10, 2015, from *www.ecfr.gov/cgi-bin/text-idx?SID=32ee40bd991b2da4d3b7bb405610f150&mc=true&node=se42.3.414_11&rgn=div8;.*

42 *CFR* §414.210 - General payment rules. (2011). Retrieved August 10, 2015, from *www.gpo.gov/fdsys/granule/CFR-2011-title42-vol3/CFR-2011-title42-vol3-sec414-210.*

42 *CFR* 416.2. - Definitions. (2010). Retrieved August 10, 2015, from *www.gpo.gov/fdsys/granule/CFR-2010-title42- vol3/ CFR- 2010-title42-vol3-sec416-2.*

42 *CFR* 416.40. Condition for coverage-Compliance with State licensure law. (2012). Retrieved August 10, 2015, from *www.gpo.gov/fdsys/granule/CFR-2012-title42-vol3/CFR-2012-title42-vol3-sec416-40.*

42 *CFR* Part 418, Subpart C - Conditions of Participation: Patient care. (2011). Retrieved August 10, 2015, from *www.gpo.gov/fdsys/pkg/CFR-2011-title42-vol3/pdf/CFR-2011-title42-vol3-part418.pdf.*

42 *CFR* §418.3 - Definitions. (2014). Retrieved August 10, 2015, from *www.gpo.gov/fdsys/pkg/CFR-2014-title42-vol3/pdf/CFR-2014-title42-vol3-sec418-3.pdf.*

42 *CFR* Part 418, Subpart G - Payment for hospice care. (2011). Retrieved August 10, 2015, from *www.gpo.gov/fdsys/pkg/CFR-2011-title42-vol3/pdf/CFR-2011-title42-vol3-part418.pdf.*

42 *CFR* 419.1 et seq. (2015). Retrieved August 10, 2015, from *www.ecfr.gov/cgi-bin/text-idx?SID=b8472aa0c41b2306621e5c388af36cd3&mc=true&node=se42.3.419_11&rgn=div8.*

42 *CFR* §424.32(b) - Requirements for comprehensive outpatient rehabilitation facility (CORF) services. (2012). Retrieved August 10, 2015, from *www.gpo.gov/fdsys/pkg/CFR-2012-title42-vol3/pdf/CFR-2012-title42-vol3-sec424-32.pdf.*

42 *CFR* §424.520(b) - Effective date of Medicare billing privilege. (2011). Retrieved August 10, 2015, from *www.gpo.gov/fdsys/pkg/CFR-2011-title42-vol3/pdf/CFR-2011-title42-vol3-sec424-520.pdf.*

42 *CFR* §424.57 - Special payment rules for items furnished by DMEPOS suppliers and issuance of DMEPOS supplier billing privileges. (2014). Retrieved August 10, 2015, from *www.gpo.gov/fdsys/pkg/CFR-2014-title42-vol3/pdf/CFR-2014-title42-vol3-sec424-57.pdf.*

42 *CFR* §482.12 - Condition of participation: Governing body. (2011). Retrieved August 10, 2015, from *www.gpo.gov/fdsys/pkg/CFR-2011-title42-vol5/pdf/CFR-2011-title42-vol5-sec482-12.pdf.*

42 *CFR* §482.21 - Condition of participation: Quality assessment and performance improvement program. (2011). Retrieved August 10, 2015, from *www.gpo.gov/fdsys/granule/CFR-2011-title42-vol5/CFR-2011-title42-vol5-sec 482-21.*

42 *CFR* §482.22 - Condition of participation: Medical staff. (2011). Retrieved August 10, 2015, from *www.gpo.gov/fdsys/granule/CFR-2011-title42-vol5/CFR-2011-title42-vol5-sec482-22.*

42 *CFR* §482.24(b) - Condition of participation: Medical record services. (2011). Retrieved August 10, 2015, from *www.gpo.gov/fdsys/granule/CFR-2011-title42-vol5/CFR-2011-title42-vol5-sec482-24.*

42 *CFR* §483, Subpart B - Requirements for long-term care facilities. (2011). Retrieved June 9, 2015, from *www.gpo.gov/fdsys/pkg/CFR-2011-title42-vol5/pdf/CFR-2011-title42-vol5-part483.pdf.*

42 *CFR* §482.26 - Condition of participation: Radiologic services. (2011). Retrieved August 10, 2015, from *www.gpo.gov/fdsys/granule/CFR-2011-title42-vol5/CFR-2011-title42-vol5-sec482-26.*

42 *CFR* §482.53 - Condition of participation: Nuclear medicine services. (1999). Retrieved August 10, 2015, from *www.gpo.gov/fdsys/granule/CFR-1999-title42-vol3/CFR-1999-title42-vol3-sec482-53.*

42 *CFR* §484.14 - Condition of participation: Organization, services, and administration. (2011). Retrieved June 9, 2015, from *www.gpo.gov/fdsys/granule/CFR-2011-title42-vol5/CFR-2011-title42-vol5-sec484-14.*

42 *CFR* §484.16 - Condition of participation: Group of professional personnel. (2011). Retrieved August 10, 2015, from *www.gpo.gov/fdsys/granule/CFR-2011-title42-vol5/CFR-2011-title42-vol5-sec484-16.*

42 *CFR* §484.18. (2007). Retrieved August 10, 2015, from *www.gpo.gov/fdsys/pkg/CFR-2007-title42-vol4/pdf/CFR-2007-title42-vol4-sec484-18.pdf.*

42 *CFR* §§484.30–38 - Condition of participation: Skilled nursing services. (2011). Retrieved August 10, 2015, from *www.gpo.gov/fdsys/granule/CFR-2011-title42-vol5/CFR-2011-title42-vol5-sec484-30.*

42 *CFR* §484.48 - Condition of participation: Clinical records. (2011). Retrieved August 10, 2015, from *www.gpo.gov/fdsys/granule/CFR-2011-title42-vol5/CFR-2011-title42-vol5-sec484-48/content-detail.html.*

42 *CFR* §485.51 - Definition. (2011). Retrieved August 10, 2015, from *www.gpo.gov/fdsys/granule/CFR-2011-title42-vol5/CFR-2011-title42-vol5-sec485-51.*

42 *CFR* 488.301 - Definitions. (2011). Retrieved June 9, 2015, from *www.gpo.gov/fdsys/granule/CFR-2011-title42-vol5/CFR-2011-title42-vol5-sec488-301.*

42 *CFR* §489.10(b) - Basic requirements. (2003). Retrieved August 10, 2015, from *www.gpo.gov/fdsys/granule/CFR-2003-title42-vol3/CFR-2003-title42-vol3-sec489-10.*

42 *CFR* §§489.20 - Basic commitments. (2010). Retrieved August 10, 2015, from *www.gpo.gov/fdsys/granule/CFR-2010-title42-vol5/CFR-2010-title42-vol5-sec489-20.*

43 *CFR* §489.24(b) - Special responsibilities of Medicare hospitals in emergency cases. (2014). Retrieved August 10, 2015, from *www.gpo.gov/fdsys/pkg/CFR-2014-title42-vol5/pdf/CFR-2014-title42-vol5-sec489-24.pdf.*

42 *CFR* §494.10 - Definitions. (2011). Retrieved August 10, 2015, from *www.gpo.gov/fdsys/granule/CFR-2011-title42-vol5/ CFR-2011-title42-vol5-sec494-10.*

42 *CFR* Part 498 - Appeals procedures for determinations that affect participation in the Medicare program and for determinations that affect the participation of ICFs/MR and certain NFs in the Medicaid program. (2011). Retrieved August 10, 2015, from *www.gpo.gov/fdsys/granule/CFR-2011-title42-vol5/CFR- 2011-title 42-vol5-part498.*

42 *USC* §1320a–7k(d) - Medicare and Medicaid program integrity provisions. (2010). Retrieved August 10, 2015, from *www.gpo.gov/fdsys/pkg/USCODE-2010-title42/pdf/USCODE-2010-title42-chap7-subchapXI-partA- sec1320a-7k.pdf.*

42 *USC* §1395x(b)(3) - Definitions. (2011). Retrieved August 10, 2015, from *www.gpo.gov/fdsys/granule/USCODE-2010-title42/USCODE-2010-title42-chap7-subchapXVIII-partE-sec1395x.*

42 *USC* §1395x(w) - Definitions. (2011). Retrieved August 10, 2015, from *www.gpo.gov/fdsys/granule/USCODE-2010-title42/USCODE-2010-title42-chap7-subchapXVIII-partE-sec1395x.*

42 *USC* 1395w–4. (n.d.). Retrieved August 10, 2015, from *www.ssa.gov/OP_Home/ssact/title18/1848.htm.*

63 *Fed. Reg.* 47552, 47588. (1998). Retrieved August 10, 2015, from *www.gpo.gov/fdsys/pkg/FR-1998-09-08/pdf/98-23383.pdf.*

65 *Fed. Reg.* 18434, 18511. (2000). Retrieved August 10, 2015, from *www.gpo.gov/fdsys/pkg/FR-2000-04-07/pdf/00-8215.pdf#page=1.*

65 *Fed. Reg.* 18434, 18515–16. (2000). Retrieved August 10, 2015, from *www.gpo.gov/fdsys/pkg/FR-2000-04-07/pdf/00-8215.pdf#page=1.*

65 *Fed. Reg.* 18504. (2000). Retrieved August 10, 2015, from *www.gpo.gov/fdsys/pkg/FR-2000-04-07/pdf/00-8215.pdf.*

65 *Fed. Reg.* 18506. (2000). Retrieved August 10, 2015, from *www.gpo.gov/fdsys/pkg/FR-2000-04-07/pdf/00-8215.pdf.*

67 *Fed. Reg.* 49982. (2002). Retrieved August 10, 2015, from *www.gpo.gov/fdsys/pkg/FR-2002-08-01/html/02-19292.htm.*

67 *Fed. Reg.* 50091. (2002). Retrieved August 10, 2015, from *www.gpo.gov/fdsys/pkg/FR-2002-08-01/html/02-19292.htm.*

68 *Fed. Reg.* 46036, 46063. (2003). Retrieved August 10, 2015, from *www.gpo.gov/fdsys/pkg/FR-2003-08-04/pdf/03-19677.pdf.*

70 *Fed. Reg.* 4858 - Office of the Inspector General, OIG Supplemental Compliance Program Guidance for Hospitals. (2005). Retrieved August 10, 2015, from *https://oig.hhs.gov/fraud/docs/complianceguidance/012705HospSupplementalGuidance.pdf.*

72 *Fed. Reg.* 66580, 66805. (2007). Retrieved August 10, 2015, from *www.cms.gov/Regulations-and-Guidance/Regulations-and-Policies/QuarterlyProviderUpdates/Downloads/cms1392fc.pdf.*

76 *Fed. Reg.* 74122, 74369–70. (2011). Retrieved August 10, 2015, from *www.gpo.gov/fdsys/pkg/FR-2011-11-30/pdf/2011-28612.pdf#page=249.*

76 *Fed. Reg.* 74122, 74,370–71. (2011). Retrieved August 10, 2015, from *www.gpo.gov/fdsys/pkg/FR-2011-11-30/pdf/2011-28612.pdf#page=250.*

78 *Fed. Reg.* 43534, 43627. (2013). Retrieved August 10, 2015, from *www.gpo.gov/fdsys/pkg/FR-2013-07-19/pdf/2013-16555.pdf.*

78 *Fed. Reg.* 50496, 50744. (2013). Retrieved August 10, 2015, from *www.federalregister.com/Browse/Document/usa/na/fr/2013/8/19/2013-18956.*

79 *Fed. Reg.* 61314, 61317. (2014). Retrieved August 10, 2015, from *www.gpo.gov/fdsys/pkg/FR-2014-10-10/pdf/2014-24248.pdf.*

79 *Fed. Reg.* 66770, 66910. (2014). Retrieved August 10, 2015, from *www.gpo.gov/fdsys/pkg/FR-2014-11-10/pdf/2014-26146.pdf.*

79 *Fed. Reg.* 66770, 66914. (2014). Retrieved August 10, 2015, from *www.gpo.gov/fdsys/pkg/FR-2014-11-10/pdf/2014-26146.pdf.*

Atkinson, G. (2009). State hospital rate-setting revisited. *Commonwealth Fund Pub.* 1332(69).

Centers for Medicare and Medicaid Services. (n.d.). CMS frequently asked questions 2297. Retrieved August 10, 2015, from *https://questions.cms.gov/faq.php?id=5005&faqId=2297.*

Centers for Medicare and Medicaid Services. (2014). Chapter 1: Inpatient hospital. *Medicare Benefit Policy Manual.* Retrieved August 10, 2015, from *www.cms.gov/Regulations-and-Guidance/Guidance/Manuals/downloads/bp102c01.pdf.*

 © 2015 HCPro

Centers for Medicare and Medicaid Services. (2014). Chapter 15: Covered medical and other health services. *Medicare Benefit Policy Manual.* Retrieved August 10, 2015, from *www.cms.gov/Regulations-and-Guidance/ Guidance/Manuals/downloads/bp102c15.pdf.*

Centers for Medicare and Medicaid Services. (2014). Chapter 6: Hospital services covered under part B. *Medicare Benefit Policy Manual.* Retrieved August 10, 2015, from *www.cms.gov/Regulations-and-Guidance/ Guidance/Manuals/downloads/bp102c06.pdf.*

Centers for Medicare and Medicaid Services. (2015). Chapter 7: Home health services. *Medicare Benefit Policy Manual.* Retrieved August 10, 2015, from *www.cms.gov/Regulations-and-Guidance/Guidance/Manuals/ downloads/bp102c07.pdf.*

Centers for Medicare and Medicaid Services. (2014). Chapter 3: Inpatient hospital. *Medicare Claims Processing Manual.* Retrieved August 10, 2015, from *www.cms.gov/Regulations-and-Guidance/Guidance/Manuals/ downloads/clm104c03.pdf.*

Centers for Medicare and Medicaid Services. (2015). Chapter 4, part B: Hospital. *Medicare Claims Processing Manual.* Retrieved August 10, 2015, from *www.cms.gov/Regulations-and-Guidance/Guidance/Manuals/ Downloads/clm104c04.pdf.*

Centers for Medicare and Medicaid Services. (2015). Chapter 5, part B: Outpatient rehabilitation and CORF/ OPT services. *Medicare Claims Processing Manual.* Retrieved from *www.cms.gov/Regulations-and-Guidance/Guidance/Manuals/downloads/clm104c05.pdf.*

Centers for Medicare and Medicaid Services. (2014). (2014). Chapter 12: Physicians/nonphysician practitioners. *Medicare Claims Processing Manual.* Retrieved August 10, 2015, from *www.cms.gov/Regulations-and-Guidance/Guidance/Manuals/Downloads/clm104c12.pdf.*

Centers for Medicare and Medicaid Services. (2014). Chapter 14: Ambulatory surgical centers. *Medicare Claims Processing Manual.* Retrieved August 10, 2015, from *www.cms.gov/Regulations-and-Guidance/Guidance/Manuals/downloads/clm104c14.pdf.*

Centers for Medicare and Medicaid Services. (2015). Chapter 23: Fee schedule administration and coding. *Medicare Claims Processing Manual.* Retrieved August 10, 2015, from *www.cms.gov/Regulations-and-Guidance/Guidance/Manuals/downloads/clm104c23.pdf.*

Centers for Medicare and Medicaid Services. (2014). Chapter 26: Completing and processing. *Medicare Claims Processing Manual.* Retrieved August 10, 2015, from *www.cms.gov/Regulations-and-Guidance/ Guidance/Manuals/downloads/clm104c26.pdf.*

Centers for Medicare and Medicaid Services. (2013). *Transmittal 2845. Medicare Claims Processing Manual.* Retrieved August 10, 2015, from *www.cms.gov/Regulations-and-Guidance/Guidance/Transmittals/ Downloads/R2845CP.pdf.*

Centers for Medicare and Medicaid Services. (2009). Chapter 5: Definitions. *Medicare General Information and Eligibility Manual.* Retrieved August 10, 2015, from *www.cms.gov/Regulations-and-Guidance/Guidance/ Manuals/Downloads/ge101c05.pdf.*

Centers for Medicare and Medicaid Services. (2009). Chapter 5: Definitions. *General Information and Eligibility Manual.* Retrieved August 10, 2015, from *www.cms.gov/Regulations-and-Guidance/Guidance/Manuals/ downloads/ge101c05.pdf.*

Denial of hospital off-site location. (2011). Retrieved August 10, 2015, from *www.isheweb.org/emails/10-3-11/ CMS-Denial-Letter.pdf.*

General Assembly of Maryland. (n.d.). Annotated code of Maryland health-general article, §19-201, et seq. Retrieved from *http://mgaleg.maryland.gov/webmga/frmStatutesText.aspx?pid= &tab=subject5&stab= &ys=2015RS&article=ghg&section=19-201&ext=html&session=2015RS*.

Hospital isn't shy about getting its take. (2014). *LA Times*. Retrieved August 10, 2015, from *www.latimes.com/ business/la-fi-lazarus-20140606-column.html*.

Hospital outpatient therapeutic services that have been evaluated for a change in supervision level. (2015). Retrieved August 10, 2015, from *www.cms.gov/Medicare/Medicare-Fee-for-Service-Payment/Hospital OutpatientPPS/Downloads/Hospital-Outpatient-Therapeutic-Services.pdf*.

In the Case of Mira Vista, Inc. (2007). *DAB Appellate Division, DAB Docket No. A-06-114*. Retrieved August 10, 2015, from *www.hhs.gov/dab/decisions/RULDAB2007-3.pdf*.

In the Case of Shady Grove Adventist Hospital Emergency Center at Germantown. (2008). *DAB Decision No. CR1783*. Retrieved August 10, 2015, from *www.hhs.gov/dab/decisions/civildecisions/2008/CR1783.pdf*.

In the Case of St. Vincent's Catholic Medical Centers of New York. (2008). *DAB Decision No. CR1734*. Retrieved August 10, 2015, from *www.hhs.gov/dab/decisions/civildecisions/2008/CR1734.pdf*.

Incorrect place-of-service claims resulted in potential Medicare overpayments costing millions. (2015). Retrieved August 10, 2015, from *https://oig.hhs.gov/oas/reports/region1/11300506.pdf*.

Medicare Payment Policy (2015). *Report to the Congress*. Retrieved August 10, 2015, from *www.medpac.gov/ documents/reports/mar2015_entirereport_revised.pdf?sfvrsn=0*.

MedPAC comment on CMS's proposed rule entitled: Medicare Program; Revisions to Payment Policies under the Physician Fee Schedule, Clinical Laboratory Fee Schedule, Access to Identifiable Data for the CMMI Models & Other Revisions for Part B for CY 2015. (2014). Retrieved August 10, 2015, from *www.medpac.gov/ documents/comment-letters/08282014_comment_letter_2015_pt_b_rule_final.pdf?sfvrsn=0*.

Mercy Hospital Lebanon. (2014). *DAB Decision No. CR3320*. Retrieved August 10, 2015, from *www.hhs.gov/dab/decisions/civildecisions/2014/cr3320.pdf*.

Office of Inspector General, U.S. Department of Health and Human Services. (1999). Hospital ownership of physician practices, OEI-05-98-00110. (1999). Retrieved from August 10, 2015, from *https://oig.hhs.gov/oei/ reports/oei-05-98-00110.pdf*.

Office of Inspector General, U.S. Department of Health and Human Services. (2014). *Work plan 2014 fiscal year*. (2014). Retrieved August 10, 2015, from *http://oig.hhs.gov/reports-and-publications/archives/workplan/ 2014/Work-Plan-2014.pdf*.

Office of Inspector General, U.S. Department of Health and Human Services. (2015). *Work plan 2015 fiscal year*. Retrieved August 10, 2015, from *http://oig.hhs.gov/reports-and-publications/archives/workplan/2015/ FY15-Work-Plan.pdf*.

Provider-based rules trigger 2nd hospital settlement; CMS targets shared space. (2015). *AIS Health*. Retrieved August 10, 2015, from *http://aishealth.com/archive/rmc040615-01*.

Public Law 106-554. (2000). Retrieved August 10, 2015, from *www.gpo.gov/fdsys/pkg/PLAW-106publ554/ pdf/PLAW-106publ554.pdf*.

Review of Place of Service Coding for Physician Services (2005). Trailblazer Health Enterprises, LLC for the period January 1, 2001 through December 31, 2002, A-06-04-00046. Retrieved August 10, 2015, from *https://oig.hhs.gov/oas/reports/region6/60400046.pdf*.

Rising hospital employment of physicians: Better quality, higher costs? (2011). *Health System Change*. Retrieved August 10, 2015, from *www.hschange.com/CONTENT/1230*.

Settlement Agreement Between United States of America and Our Lady of Lourdes Memorial Hospital. (2014). Retrieved August 10, 2015, from *www.kslaw.com/library/newsletters/healthheadlines/2014/1020/ hh102014_Lourdes.pdf.*

Shady Grove Adventist Hospital. (2008). *Appellate Division Decision No. 2221.* Retrieved August 10, 2015, from *www.hhs.gov/dab/decisions/dabdecisions/dab2221.pdf.*

Social Security Act §1819(a). (n.d.) Requirements for, and assuring quality of care in, skilled nursing facilities. Retrieved August 10, 2015, from *www.ssa.gov/OP_Home/ssact/title18/1819.htm.*

Social Security Act §1861(dd)(1). (n.d.) Miscellaneous provisions. Retrieved August 10, 2015, from *www. socialsecurity.gov/OP_Home/ssact/title18/1861.htm.*

The Physicians' Hospital In Anadarko. (2006). *DAB Decision No. CR1460.* Retrieved August 10, 2015, from *www.hhs.gov/dab/decisions/CR1460.htm.*

Transmittal A-03-030. (2003). Provider-based status on or after October 1, 2002. Retrieved August 10, 2015, from *www.cms.gov/Regulations-and-Guidance/Guidance/Transmittals/downloads/A03030.pdf.*

Transmittal 3315. (2015). New and revised place of service codes (POS) for outpatient hospital. Retrieved August 10, 2015, from *www.cms.gov/Regulations-and-Guidance/Guidance/Transmittals/Downloads/ R3315CP.pdf.*

Union Hospital, Inc. (2011). *DAB Decision No. CR2422.* Retrieved August 10, 2015, from *www.hhs.gov/dab/ decisions/civildecisions/2011/cr2422.pdf.*

West Virginia Code. (n.d.). Chapter 16, §16-29B-1 et seq. Retrieved August 10, 2015, from *www.legis.state.wv.us/wvcode/ChapterEntire.cfm?chap=16&art=29&section=1.*

Why you might pay twice for one visit to a doctor. (2012). *Seattle Times.* Retrieved August 10, 2015, from *www.seattletimes.com/seattle-news/why-you-might-pay-twice-for-one-visit-to-doctor/.*